PRAISE FOR DARK

"Part scholar, part journalist, part wide-eyed death enthusiast, Rosenbloom takes readers on her own journey to understand how and why human-skin books came to be . . . She includes no shortage of memorable scientific minutiae and clarifications of misunderstood history along the way."

—James Hamblin, *The New York Times Book Review*
(Editors' Choice)

"Against all odds, a delight . . . Regardless of how wacky or tragic any particular book's journey has been, Rosenbloom approaches them all with such good humor, solid science, and unerring respect for the dead that *Dark Archives* manages to be life-affirming amidst all the ethical debate and stinky tannery mishaps."

—Emma Grey Ellis, *Wired*

"[*Dark Archives*] begins as a quest for the fascinating and forbidden: the reader is invited to share the thrill of pursuit, and of the moment when the sinister and legendary provenance of a book is scientifically verified. But as the histories of these books unfold, the focus necessarily shifts from their creators and possessors to the lives of those who supplied the skin."

—Mike Jay, *The New York Review of Books*

"What begins as an investigation into fascinatingly macabre volumes becomes a reflection on medical ethics, consent and mortality."

—*The Economist*

"An engaging chronicle of a shadowy aspect of clinical medicine . . . Despite the grisly nature of the proceedings, *Dark Archives* succeeds precisely because Rosenbloom respects the books for their research value as well as the people whose skin was used to bind them, often without their consent."

—Frank Brasile, *Shelf Awareness*

"As Rosenbloom crisscrosses the globe to confirm the purported origins of skin-bound books—a cracking detective story in itself—her journey offers unusual insight into what defines informed consent, what separates homage from exploitation, and how power disparities can breed casual inhumanity."

—Elizabeth Svoboda, *Undark*

"Meticulously researched and ceaselessly fascinating...Rosenbloom, being an affable and magnetic narrator, takes readers on a journey from libraries to museums and private collectors...*Dark Archives* deftly ties the macabre together with the educational and amusing."

—Jonathan Peltz, *L.A. Taco*

"How do you sum up a brilliant writer, an intensely unique and intriguing subject matter, and one of the coolest, most thrillingly researched books you've ever read...in a way that isn't massively hyperbolic or, conversely, somehow doesn't do any of it enough justice?...[Rosenbloom] doesn't just detail these books, or the collectors, or the people who created them; she passionately and humanely explores *the people* they used to be...Come for the weird book facts, stay for the unexpected and powerful human questions."

—S. Elizabeth, *Haute Macabre*

"Reminiscent of Mary Roach, Rosenbloom's tone is inquisitive and, at turns, morbidly funny and deeply contemplative...We can revel with a morbid gaze at the strangeness of anthropodermic books, but Rosenbloom's investigation forces readers to reflect on our own relationship to medicine and exploitation of the dead."

—Marisa Mercurio, *Sublime Horror*

"Wide-ranging, engagingly written, and unusual...[*Dark Archives*] will fascinate those interested in a new angle from which to consider what it means to be human and what our responsibilities are to other people...Essential."

—Stephanie Klose, *Library Journal* (starred review)

"Fascinating . . . Rosenbloom's conversational tone and obvious excitement at the thrill of the chase counterbalances the macabre nature of her subject . . . This unique and well-researched account shines an intriguing light on a hidden corner of the rare books world."   —*Publishers Weekly*

"[An] intriguing intersection of history, science, and the macabre . . . A unique conversation about consent, medical ethics, and legalities . . . Rosenbloom's passion for the topic is infused in each page, making for a captivating read."   —Michelle Ross, *Booklist*

"Profoundly odd, wholly original, and utterly engrossing! If 'Who Knew?' were a Pulitzer category, Megan Rosenbloom's *Dark Archives* would win it hands down."
                             —Erik Larson, author of *The Splendid and the Vile: A Saga of Churchill, Family, and Defiance During the Blitz*

"*Dark Archives* is a gorgeous dive into the humanity and inhumanity of the people behind (and on) these strangely captivating books. Propelled by curiosity and bibliophilia, Megan Rosenbloom travels far and wide and deep within, taking us to unimaginable places. This is a masterful work, enlightened and enlivened by Rosenbloom's scholarship and her involvement with the death-positive movement. If there were a word for the perfect pairing of author and subject and the giddy joy that pairing brings to the reader, I'd be using it right now."
                             —Mary Roach, author of *Grunt: The Curious Science of Humans at War*

"An international treasure hunt, a fascinating medical history, a high-level PR nightmare, and a heartrending account of the real people whose flesh was turned into curiosities by the medical professionals they trusted."
                             —Caitlin Doughty, author of *Will My Cat Eat My Eyeballs? Big Questions from Tiny Mortals About Death*

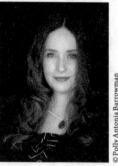

MEGAN ROSENBLOOM

DARK ARCHIVES

Megan Rosenbloom is a librarian with a research interest in the history of medicine and rare books. Formerly a medical librarian and journalist, she is now the collection strategies librarian at UCLA Library in Los Angeles. She is also the president of the Southern California Society for the History of Medicine. She is a member of the Anthropodermic Book Project, a multidisciplinary team scientifically testing alleged human skin books around the world to verify their human origin. A proponent of the death-positive movement, she was also the cofounder and director of Death Salon, the events arm of the Order of the Good Death.

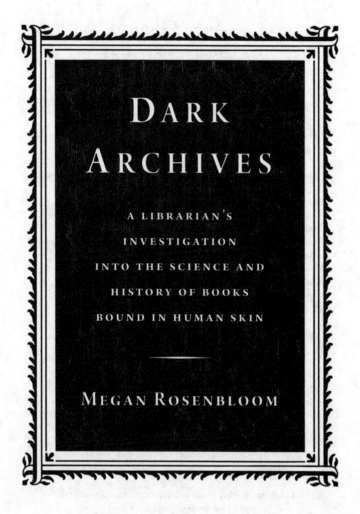

DARK ARCHIVES

A LIBRARIAN'S INVESTIGATION INTO THE SCIENCE AND HISTORY OF BOOKS BOUND IN HUMAN SKIN

MEGAN ROSENBLOOM

PICADOR

FARRAR, STRAUS AND GIROUX   NEW YORK

Picador
120 Broadway, New York 10271

Printed in the United States of America
Originally published in 2020 by Farrar, Straus and Giroux
First paperback edition, 2021

Photograph of Hans Holbein's *The Dance of Death* (London: Chiswick
Press, 1898), courtesy of John Hay Library, Brown University.

The Library of Congress has cataloged the Farrar, Straus and Giroux
hardcover edition as follows:
Names: Rosenbloom, Megan, 1981– author.
Title: Dark archives : a librarian's investigation into the science and
history of books bound in human skin / Megan Rosenbloom.
Description: First edition. | New York : Farrar, Straus and Giroux, 2020. |
Includes bibliographical references and index.
Identifiers: LCCN 2020023645 | ISBN 9780374134709 (hardcover)
Subjects: LCSH: Anthropodermic books.
Classification: LCC Z269.3.A58 R67 2020 | DDC 002—dc23
LC record available at https://lccn.loc.gov/2020023645

Paperback ISBN: 978-1-250-80016-9

Designed by Gretchen Achilles

Our books may be purchased in bulk for promotional, educational, or
business use. Please contact your local bookseller or the Macmillan
Corporate and Premium Sales Department at 1-800-221-7945, extension 5442, or
by email at MacmillanSpecialMarkets@macmillan.com.

For book club information, please visit facebook.com/picadorbookclub or
email marketing@picadorusa.com.

picadorusa.com · instagram.com/picador
twitter.com/picadorusa · facebook.com/picadorusa

3   5   7   9   10   8   6   4

For Cathy Curran, whose bravery, strength,
and sense of humor inspired me to write this book.
Now you *have* to read it, Mom.

Contents

Author's Note.. ix

Prologue: Under Glass... 3

1. The First Printing....................................... 19

2. This Dreadful Workshop 35

3. Gentlemen Collectors 49

4. Skin Craft 67

5. Secrets of the Sages-Femmes 79

6. The Long Shadow of the Night Doctors 95

7. The Postmortem Travels of William Corder 115

8. Echoes of Tanner's Close.............................131

9. The Highwayman's Gift 147

10. Ghosts in the Library 161

11. My Corpse, My Choice............................ 185

12. The French Connection 197

Epilogue: Humane Anatomy 211

The Anthropodermic Book Project's List of Confirmed
Human Skin Books as of March 2020 229

Notes.. 231

Acknowledgments...259

Index 263

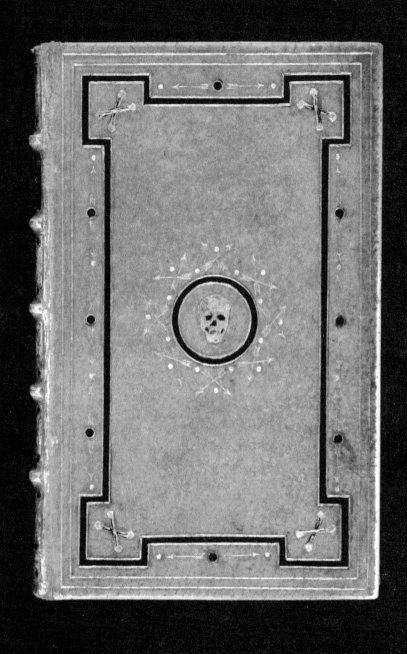

Author's Note

Regarding the Anthropodermic Book Project's scientific testing results, the project's data is not currently shared publicly, so where possible I cite our results as they have been reported in a publicly available place—in news media or a library catalog, for instance. In cases where our peptide mass fingerprinting results have not been reported publicly elsewhere, any conclusions I share in this book have been endorsed by the institutions.

I have included just one image of a confirmed anthropodermic book: an 1898 copy of Hans Holbein's *The Dance of Death* from Brown University's John Hay Library. I chose to share this image because I find it to be the most beautiful of the anthropodermic books and the most artfully bound. Unlike the *Necronomicon* or the spellbook in Disney's 1993 film *Hocus Pocus*, real human skin books do not usually immediately announce themselves with a ghoulish appearance. They do not look much different from any other antiquarian book you would find on the shelf. It's likely some are quietly resting in library stacks, hiding in plain sight. Even if you were holding one right now, you probably wouldn't be able to tell.

DARK
ARCHIVES

UNDER GLASS

The brass, wood, and glass cases gave the main exhibition hall of the Mütter Museum a warm and cozy feeling—which was odd, considering it was a room full of corpses. It was 2008, and I was in library school and working for a medical publisher. Often, after a docent shift at the nearby Rosenbach museum, I strolled through this world-renowned collection of medical oddities. Each time, I noticed something new or saw a familiar specimen in a different way. One day, I might linger in front of the liver shared by Chang and Eng Bunker (known as the original "Siamese Twins"); another I would marvel at a human colon longer than my car. The Mütter Museum of the College of Physicians of Philadelphia is the kind of place that encourages a mix of eager fascination and quiet contemplation of mortality.

On the second floor stood an inconspicuous glass display case featuring leather-bound books. As a library school student who was falling in love with rare books, I found it peculiar to see a row of them displayed with their covers closed. When I noticed the captions inside the cases, I gasped and looked around, as if to find some passerby to corroborate what I was seeing. The text claimed that these books—and an accompanying leather wallet—were made from human skin.

As I read on, I was even more shocked to learn that doctors once made these skin books as luxury items for their private rare book collections. There was one doctor, Joseph Leidy, whose personal copy of his book, *An Elementary Treatise on Human Anatomy*, was bound in the skin of a Civil War soldier patient. In the letter that accompanied the book's donation to the museum, Leidy's descendant called it a "most cherished possession."

I could imagine a serial killer making objects from human remains and keeping them as trophies. But a doctor? Was there a time when this practice was acceptable, when doctors could do this with their patients' bodies? Most people today would assume that if a doctor did something so ghoulish, it must have happened during the Nazi era. But as I would later discover, there were no known human skin books from that time. Unlike the other human remains on display at the Mütter, these books with their covers closed could not teach medical students about rare diseases or conditions they might never be able to encounter at a patient's bedside. A dead person's skin had become a by-product of the dissection process, like a piece of animal leather after a butcher's slaughter, harvested solely to make a doctor's personal books more collectible and valuable. The fifty-cent phrase for this practice is anthropodermic bibliopegy: a combination of the Greek root words for human (*anthropos*), skin (*derma*), book (*biblion*), and fasten (*pegia*).

The implications of all this unfurled as I tried to put myself in the shoes of the respectable doctor bibliophile who would create such a monstrosity. Rare book collectors thrill at the unique specimen, as do I. But the ways in which many rare book collectors evaluate a book are surface level only: its age, its wear, the beauty of its illustrations, the ornamentation of its binding, and yes, of course, the nature of the content contained in its physical package. Looking at an anthropodermic book from this kind of bibliophilic viewpoint, the allure builds: it is far more expensive now, the material is rarer; perhaps there is a juicy provenance story that I can share with friends over drinks in the den, when I trot out my unusual treasure for them to see. But that's the point where my imaginary bibliophile loses me. Those just could not be good enough reasons for creating books out of other humans.

From a more humanistic perspective, the interest in these strange books doesn't fade, but becomes far richer. What were the circumstances in the life of the author responsible for the creation of a text someone saw fit to bind in human skin? Who were the people depicted in these anatomical illustrations? Who supplied the skin that was used for this anthropodermic book, and how did this fate befall them? Who were the binders who agreed to put the skin on the book, and who were the collectors who commissioned the anthropodermic bindings? Through whose hands did this book pass before it came to its current home at the College of Physicians of Philadelphia, and what context did each owner bring to the book and its history? Who are the stewards at these institutions who keep the book safe for future scholars, and who are those scholars that find their way to that book and interrogate it with their own special lenses? Whose stories am I missing altogether? When I rehumanize these books, suddenly the scores of human beings whom each book has touched cluster in my mind's eye like a community together holding one small object. That was the story I wanted to know. That was the story I wanted to tell.

I never would have guessed that a lineup of innocent-looking books in a glass museum case would take over my life.

THE NOVEMBER SUN winked through my dirty car window as I rolled past the orange groves that line the entrance to the Huntington in San Marino, California. It was now 2015 and I was the librarian in charge of the medical collections at the University of Southern California. I nodded to the attendant and found my favorite parking spot. My Saturday morning ritual as a reader in the research library was beginning to feel pleasantly familiar. Most people know these idyllic grounds as the Huntington Gardens instead of by their full name (the Huntington Library, Art Museum, and Botanical Gardens), which is understandable given the estate's astounding 120 acres of manicured greenery. Even though it's right there in the name, most visitors seem to have no idea there's a world-class library and research center in the midst of this paradise. Even my local friends have told me they have never been inside the buildings at the Huntington that display for the public rare books, artifacts from throughout the history of science, and fine art collections. Fewer still notice the massive Munger Research Center, despite its location near the front entrance. Every day, throngs of visitors coast right past the columned building on their way to the gardens with their strollers and cameras in tow. Their loss.

The white Munger building always felt like an iceberg to me, with its many floors underground housing a staggering eleven million items spanning ten centuries. Sometimes I would get hopelessly, pleasurably lost in its labyrinthine open stacks with nothing but a call number penciled on a piece of paper. More often I waited in the cushy reading room, gazing from bust to bust at the stony faces of the intellectual luminaries that line the walls, until a page retrieved my requested volume from the unfathomable depths. Another attendant would hand it to me and I would deposit it on a velvet book cradle that positions it for reading but puts less stress on the binding than opening it flat. The Huntington is one of the greatest independent research libraries in the world, but let's face it: it's the gardens that hundreds of thousands flock to every year. Being a reader there feels like breaching some inner sanctum.

On my mornings there panning for bibliographic gold in, say, the scrapbook of some master bookbinder or one of Jacques d'Agoty's velvety anatomical atlases, I have felt awe and gratitude as a medical librarian to have this collection in my city, and excitement for what I might find. I had come a long way in the seven years since I first encountered human skin books at the College of Physicians of Philadelphia. No longer did glass cases separate me from the artifacts that tickled my intellectual curiosity.

As I approached this hallowed place on this particular Saturday, I confronted a feeling that was new to me: fear. My tote bag contained a manila envelope that was packed with some gloves, a handful of small, conical plastic Eppendorf Tubes, and a metal scalpel with individually sealed blades. I started to sweat, feeling like I shouldn't be allowed into the library with this contraband.

Stephen Tabor, the curator of rare books at the Huntington, was waiting for me at the security desk. We already knew each other; we're both members of the Zamorano Club, a

Southern California bibliophile society that is a convivial mix of rare book sellers, collectors, and librarians. But today there was some extra gravity in the air, because instead of coming to read the Huntington's treasures, I was there to cut them. I planned to take minute pieces of two of them away to be scientifically tested; I wanted to find out whether the objects in question had the most macabre of distinctions—being made from human skin. The samples would come from a parchment note and a medical book entitled *Anatomy Epitomized and Illustrated . . .* , an alleged example of anthropodermic bibliopegy. This minor destruction was a necessary evil if we hoped to understand these mysterious collection items in a previously unimaginable way.

Anthropodermic bibliopegy has been a specter on the shelves of libraries, museums, and private collections for over a century. Human skin books—mostly made by nineteenth-century doctor bibliophiles—are the only books that are controversial not for the ideas they contain but for the physical makeup of the object itself. They repel and fascinate, and their very ordinary appearances mask the horror inherent in their creation. Anthropodermic books tell a complicated and uncomfortable tale about the development of clinical medicine and the doctoring class, and the worst of what can come from the collision of acquisitiveness and a distanced clinical gaze. The weight of these objects' fraught legacy transfers to the institutions where they are housed, and the library and museum professionals who are responsible for them. Each owner handles this responsibility differently.

Very little is known about these books or even how many examples of this practice may exist. Often the lore surrounding anthropodermic books was passed down without any way of knowing whether they were indeed made out of human skin, and if they were, how they were created, and whose bodies they once were.

Only a year before, in 2014, after hundreds of years of whispers and allusions about anthropodermic books, the conservationists at Harvard Library had discovered that a simple scientific test could be employed to confirm definitively whether an alleged human skin book was genuine. Shortly thereafter, I joined forces with the chemist who carried out the Harvard test, another chemist, and the curator of the Mütter Museum in Philadelphia to create the Anthropodermic Book Project. Our aim is to identify and test as many alleged anthropodermic books as possible and dispel long-held myths about the most macabre books in history. Sometimes the most unlikely candidates turn out to be real human skin, and some books with plausible pedigrees turn out to be frauds. As of this writing, my team has identified only about fifty alleged anthropodermic books in public collections and a few more in private hands. With such a small field of study, any test result could completely reshape our understanding of the scope of this practice. We have to approach every item objectively and let the science out the truth.

Tabor led me to an area of the Munger building I had never seen, where his colleagues from the conservation department stood, stone-faced, around some dark leather objects on a table. I could tell they were just as uncomfortable with this situation as I was—most librarians would feel squeamish about removing pieces of antique books, regardless of the purpose. I wished I had worn something more clinical than my cheery yellow cardigan; something like a white lab coat might have been more reassuring. Little did they know that this was my first time wielding the knife.

The objects I was testing that day at the Huntington were representative of the scope of what the Anthropodermic Book Project encounters. I had done some sleuthing and found that the book *Anatomy Epitomized and Illustrated* . . . was printed in 1737 and attributed to a writer called "M.N.," who historians believe was Thomas Gibson, physician-general of the English army. Originally published in 1682, this book attempted to sum up all that was known about the structures of the human body and expanded on an even older manual compiled by dozens of anatomists. Many confirmed human skin books didn't begin their print life in this controversial binding but were rebound by collectors, usually doctors who took the oldest or rarest texts in their private collections and rebound them in skin removed from a corpse during anatomical dissection. Doctor book collectors had access to this rarest of binding material, and the resulting books became far rarer and therefore more valuable. While I had been unable thus far to identify the doctor who created this wrinkly, dark brown leather book, it was previously owned by Dr. Blake Watson, the former obstetrics department chair at St. John's Health Center in Santa Monica, California, who then donated the book to the library at the Los Angeles County Medical Association (a far less famous LACMA than the museum that also bears that acronym). This library once contained a wealth of rare medical books and had a very active user base of doctor bibliophiles who also formed a Friends of the LACMA Library society. When the library closed, the books moved to the Huntington's already formidable history of science collection, and the Friends of the LACMA group was eventually renamed the Southern California Society for the History of Medicine. The group continues to host lectures at the Huntington to this day, and I serve as their president. The provenance that I was able to uncover for *Anatomy Epitomized and Illustrated . . .* is characteristic of the way many alleged anthropodermic books pass through the hands of physician book collectors and end up in venerable institutions like the Huntington.

The other item I was sampling that day was an asymmetrical piece of parchment. It had a tawny appearance with darker patches throughout, especially around its brittle edges. With spellings and capitalizations unfamiliar in modern English (perhaps indicating illiteracy), the inscription told a harrowing tale:

> This is the skin of a White Man, taken by a Ingen, Scalped and skinned Alive belly cut out. Tied to Bed of Cols and Rosted to Deth. A White skin if took is Prise of tribe. The Ingen from Ulisses use Pale Skin for money. We Are ordered to Albeny. If we kep our skin. 117 Brave Men are lost some are sick. Genl Sullivan's ARMY. Luke Swaatland of Wyoming. Sept. 13 1779.

If true, this note pointed to a number of horrific allegations against Native Americans in New York around the American Revolution. The author not only accused them of roasting a man on a bed of coals and flaying his skin to make this piece of parchment, but also charged an entire tribe with using White skin as currency.

There was a real Luke Swetland (not Swaatland) in that era from Wyoming Valley, Pennsylvania, who was kidnapped while canoeing on the Susquehanna River on August 25, 1778. His story was relayed in 1915 by his great-grandson Edward Merrifield in the book *The Story of the Captivity and Rescue from the Indians of Luke Swetland: An Early Settler of the Wyoming Valley and a Soldier of the American Revolution.* The narrative recounts Swetland's forced travel to what is now Appleton, New York, where he became "grandson" to an elderly Native American woman and her granddaughters and did physical labor at their home. "The Indians were remarkably kind to me and made me a good many presents," wrote Swetland in a diary entry featured in the book. "In many other ways they showed me great respect."

Fourteen months after his abduction and following many botched escapes, Swetland successfully fled and returned to his family. "To them it at first seemed like an apparition," Merrifield wrote of his great-grandfather's return. "But there he truly was, in flesh and blood."

Did Swetland write this desperate note on the preserved skin of another captive? I had my doubts. The note's date struck me as too close to the date when he reunited with his family for it to have been written under immediate threat of torture. The spelling also made me a bit suspicious. Although the note was written right around the time that American English coalesced into standard, agreed-upon spellings,* Swetland's grandson claimed he was an avid reader. He would probably have had a standard spelling of his own last name (though even that is not 100 percent certain, given the time period).

While I have skills that benefit the Anthropodermic Book Project, manual dexterity is not one of them. I am by all accounts a klutz, and envisioned impaling myself with the scalpel and contaminating the Huntington samples in the process.

---

* Many credit Noah Webster, particularly his 1806 dictionary, with making the greatest advances in standardizing American English spelling.

I held my breath as I tried to remove the smallest portion of leather possible from the antique book and the parchment, deposited the miniscule flakes into capped plastic tubes, and labeled them, then sent them to the chemists on my team to analyze via peptide mass fingerprinting (PMF), the same process the Harvard Library used in 2014.

The process goes like this: First, remove a tiny chunk of a book's binding with a scalpel or sharp tweezers; if the chunk is visible to the human eye, it is more than enough. The sample is digested in an enzyme called trypsin and the mixture is dropped onto a MALDI (Matrix-Assisted Laser Desorption/Ionization) plate. The MALDI plate is placed into a mass spectrometer, where lasers irradiate the sample to identify its peptides (the short chains of amino acids that are the building blocks of proteins) and create a peptide mass fingerprint (PMF). The "fingerprint" looks like a line graph of peaks and valleys, and each fingerprint corresponds with an entry in a library of known examples from animals.

Each animal family shares a strain of protein markers that act as reference points scientists can use to distinguish one from another. As Daniel Kirby—the chemist who performed the first PMF tests on alleged anthropodermic books—explained to me, for some animal families (whales, for example) there are enough reference points and enough evolutionary variation among the species that make up a family to identify animals down to the species level. The Bovidae family of cloven-hoofed ruminants is very large, and its members share all but one of the same protein markers—but that last marker allows PMF to distinguish between sheep, goat, and cow leather, the three most common animal hides used in bookbinding. When the test is a match for the Hominidae family (known as the great apes), identifying a sample on the family level is as precise as the PMF test gets, because humans are too close in evolutionary time to the other members of the Hominidae family to have distinct protein markers from them. This imprecision might seem like a detriment, but it lends itself well to testing books bound in human skin, because if the markers match the Hominidae family, then it is almost definitely a human skin book. (I say *almost* definitely, because I have never seen or even heard of any book bound in the skin of another great ape, but reader, if you find one, do let me know.)

Collagen, one of the proteins that makes up human and animal skin, lasts far longer in an old object than DNA usually does, as long as the skin was preserved through a suitable method such as leather tanning or mummification. At the same time, processes like leather tanning often destroy much of the testable DNA remaining in an object. DNA testing can be a tricky prospect when it comes to antique books with tanned leather covers that get handled by humans, who can contaminate a sample with their own DNA. Advances in historical and ancient DNA extraction and analysis are progressing rapidly, thanks mostly to recent developments that have enabled the sequencing of many DNA molecules at once, generating large data sets that give greater insight into DNA that has been damaged by time. In the five years since our first PMF testing of human skin books, a new field called biocodicology has emerged, where the physical structures of books are studied with tools using proteins, genes, and microorganisms and their genes. This exciting work can not only tell us new facts about the books' production but offer glimpses into the old worlds where the books were created, including ancient animal husbandry practices and evidence of plague (and some poor scribe's meager lunch) on 1630 death registers. Even in the field's infancy, the results and future possibilities are enticing.

Most biocodicological studies so far have focused on parchment, which is animal skin that has been preserved by stretching, scraping, and drying but that has not been subjected to the harsh chemical processes of leather tanning. Therefore, much more of the DNA in parchment book covers or pages remains intact. Many parchment books are from the medieval era, and institutions that house them often have very strict policies regarding destructive sampling, even if the sample would barely be visible to the naked eye. Budding biocodicologists have been pioneering less destructive methods of gathering DNA from eraser rubbings on parchment—a method our team will investigate in the future to see if it works equally well in the most unusual circumstance of tanned human leather. It's always best, when working with historical artifacts, to use the methods that are the least invasive but still get the job done. For now, the most cutting-edge, next-gen DNA sequencing methods also cost more than many institutions or individual collectors can afford, whereas the cost of PMF testing is marginal to those with access to the equipment, and can be taught to conservators and curators who are not lab scientists. If these future avenues prove resistant to contamination from human handling, we might be able to learn more about the people who were made into these books, like their biological sex. In the meantime, PMF testing is a very inexpensive and reliable method for distinguishing human skin leather from other animals', and research into an individual book's provenance is our primary means of filling in historical gaps.

Being on the front lines of this intersection of history and science is nothing short of thrilling; discovering every test result feels like opening a present on Christmas morning. When we had the Huntington's PMF results in hand, they confirmed my hunches in both cases. *Anatomy Epitomized and Illustrated...* was bound in real human skin, in keeping with its medical provenance. The Swaatland note was written on cowhide.

Why would someone lie about making something of human skin? In short, money. The scarcity of an object made from human skin and the attendant morbid curiosity drive its value. The PMF result calls into question all sorts of things about the Swaatland note: Is it even from the eighteenth century, or did someone create it later on to capitalize on Swetland's captivity narrative? The item's association with such a narrative—a truly American genre that recounted harrowing tales of kidnappings, usually by people of a different race from the victim—points to a possible darker motivation. Scholars have argued that the captivity narrative helped demonize Native Americans and justify Manifest Destiny to the West. Is this note an example of that mindset in action?

Though it is unlikely that I will ever find a smoking gun—such as a letter from a human-skin-object forger that handily details the creator's motivations (I wish)—it is the ambiguity in the motivations behind the frauds that makes the fakes as intriguing to me as the real deal. Just over half of the objects we've tested so far have been made out of real human skin, so there are a great number of fakes out there. They all add a piece to the puzzle of the phenomenon of anthropodermic bibliopegy and the context in the history of medicine in which these books could be created.

Human skin books force us to consider how we approach death and illness, and what we owe to those who have been wronged or used by medical practitioners. It is my job—and my privilege—to help cultivate multiple ways of thinking about our relationships with our bodies, particularly in the context of the medical profession.

I started researching books bound in human skin because of a gut feeling that their murky histories had a lot to tell us about the price of a distanced clinical gaze. But so little was known about these macabre objects; the only mentions of them in the academic literature are old and filled with more rumor and innuendo than confirmed fact. The Internet accounts were laughably worse; for example, if you Google Images search "anthropodermic bibliopegy" you get a few real examples but mostly just a mix of odd-looking old books and the kind of obvious fake that a taxidermist, regarding a stuffed jackalope, would call a gaff. Some are clearly movie props or replicas, but others purport to be real—even when they have, say, the shadow of an actual face on the cover—and many of these creepypasta images are included in online articles about the practice as if they were genuine.*

Rare book librarians have long known that each old book is like a mystery quietly awaiting its detective: the quires, the chain lines and watermarks in the paper, the medieval sheet music hidden under bindings. Behind each step of the book's creation, there are artisans whose names are forever lost to time. I have come to understand why terms such as *bibliomania* were coined; when a detective is intrigued by a particularly nuanced case, obsession lurks just around the corner. As I hunt down the stories that attach themselves over time to these most mysterious of books, I see them less as objects and more

---

* Creepypastas are horror stories or images shared widely around the Internet, usually with no attributable author or basis in fact. Works in the genre play with the line between reality and fiction, akin to online urban legends.

as vessels for stories—the stories contained within the pages, of course, but also the stories of the people whose skin may bind the covers.

I have spent more than five years traveling to see these books for myself. Along the way, I have discovered that they provide extraordinary insight into the medical profession's complicated relationship with its past. I've also talked with colleagues to discern what these controversial objects mean for libraries today and what lessons about life and death they can hold for all of us.

This mission has taken me into some of the world's most venerable cultural institutions and smallest community museums. I've met collection custodians who are incredibly excited to have these most unusual books with their dark pedigrees accessible on their shelves. I've met others desperate to bury them—sometimes figuratively, sometimes literally in the ground. I've uncovered some fascinating historical characters—bookbinders and those they bound—and they've illuminated how those in power viewed disenfranchised people's bodies with blithe banality. Anthropodermic books demand that we wrestle with mortality and what happens when immortality is thrust upon us, and they have clarified my own moral vision as a librarian and caretaker of what remains of the past. All of these realizations came to me over time. I started off with simply a healthy dose of morbid curiosity.

THE FIRST PRINTING

Of all the reasons someone would want to go to Harvard, morbid curiosity is a rare one. Back in early 2015, I headed to Harvard's Houghton Library to see what was then the only scientifically verified anthropodermic book. Coming from a working-class background, I was astounded that simply because I was library faculty at a major research university, I could write to another university and say, "I would like to see your human skin book, please," and they would say, "Certainly, come on over." I was determined to put that extraordinary privilege to use at every opportunity. While most people scuttle with their heads down through Harvard Yard in the blustery spring winds, I am always that person lingering near the sundial that reads, "On this moment hangs eternity," my starry-eyed expression giving me away as a hopeless history nerd who is just supremely happy to get to be there.

Once inside Houghton's reading room, I removed my mittens, blew on my hands, and took Arsène Houssaye's *Des destinées de l'ame* (Destinies of the Soul) from its cradle. The outside was a mottled leather with large, visible pores. Inside, the book's endpapers were decorated with jaunty, brightly colored *L*s and *B*s (presumably the initials of its former owner, Dr. Ludovic Bouland), and two symbols associated with France and the medical profession, respectively—the fleur-de-lis and the staff of Asclepius (a snake wrapped around a rod). When I opened its pages, I read a dedication that I found unexpectedly heart-wrenching for a human skin book.

I translated it from the French as follows:

> *I dedicate this book,*
> *to you*
> *who has been the soul of this house,*
> *who calls to me in the house of God,*
> *who has left before me*
> *to make me love the path to death,*
> *you whose memory is sweet*
> *like the perfume from rivers of regret*
> *you who put children in this house,*
> *you who will never return*
> *but always have your place in this house,*
> *you who have been*
> *muse, wife, and mother*
> *with the three beauties*
> *grace, love, and virtue;*
> *to you*
> *whom I have loved, whom I love, whom I will love.*

By the 1880s, the elderly author Arsène Houssaye had turned his attention away from the drama, satire, and art criticism that had marked his writing career to ruminate on the soul, and what happens to people such as his beloved wife when their souls escape this world. Beset by grief, he delved into the philosophic, scientific, poetic, and occult conceptions of the soul, and mused about its immortality in *Des destinées de l'ame*.

He gave a copy of the work to his bibliophile friend Ludovic Bouland. Dr. Bouland had been holding on to a piece of skin from a woman's back for some years and decided it would be put to good use as a covering for his brokenhearted friend's new book. "If you look attentively you can easily distinguish the pores of the skin," Bouland marveled in a handwritten note in the front of *Des destinées de l'ame*, where its lower quality, acidic paper burned a ghostly, reverse negative image of the note on the facing page. "A book on the human soul merits that it be given human clothing."

At the Houghton Library, I held this clothing—in my bare hands, I might add. The number one question put to librarians who handle rare books is, "What, no gloves?" Wearing gloves to handle rare books actually makes you more likely to rip a page. Unless you're handling old photos on which you might leave a permanent fingerprint or touching an object that could physically harm you (and in my career, those instances do arise—thinking of you, frontier-era dental kit full of mercury and who knows what else), it is best to simply wash and dry your hands frequently when looking through rare books. Gloves are for photos—either handling them, or posing for one in which wearing the gloves makes you look like a Very Serious Researcher.

The copy of *Des destinées de l'ame* in my hands doesn't look much different from other leather-bound books of its era, except it's a bit simpler in design. Before peptide mass fingerprinting, studying the follicle patterns on the leather served as the most common method for identifying which animal supplied a book's leather. Rare book sellers still apply this method to discern the leather's animal of origin when describing books for sale. The idea is that the arrangements of human hair follicles differ from that of a cow or pig; some conservation labs put high-powered microscopes to use for this purpose. This method works for most common uses, but follicle patterns can be unreliable. During the tanning process, leather stretches and warps in unpredictable ways, so discerning a triangle pattern from a diamond shape can be rather subjective. Age can also wear away the follicle patterns. The consequences are minimal if a book dealer mistakes Morocco leather for calf. But the change in stakes and price between an animal leather book and a human leather one is substantial.

In 2014, Harvard Library had PMF tested three books from three different library locations to find out if they were human. *Des destinées de l'ame* was determined to be genuine human skin; two other alleged anthropodermic books were determined to be bound in sheepskin. One, Juan Gutiérrez's 1605 publication *Practicarum quaestionum circa leges regias Hispaniae* (loosely: Practical Questions on the Laws of Spain), was normally housed in the Harvard Law School Library, but when I visited, it was in the conservation department being repaired, so I couldn't see it. Instead, I went to the medical library to see the other fake.

When I arrived at the Countway Library of Medicine, the attendant at the rare book room desk said those magic words every researcher loves to hear: "Jack told me to tell you that he pulled a couple of surprises for you." She meant the librarian Jack Eckert, whom I had come to visit. She shuffled back to the shelf of requested materials and read aloud from the envelope. "Tattoo on human skin . . ." Her smile melted into a grimace.

I chuckled nervously. "You're probably thinking, 'What is this lady getting me into this morning?'"

"Never a dull moment," she sighed, handing me the heavy plain white envelope.

People tend to think librarians sit around reading books all day. If only. In some circumstances, the job can be surprisingly dangerous. I once had a run-in with a donated box of rare medical materials at my own library. I pawed around some wadded-up brown paper surrounding the mystery items in the box and felt a sharp prick on my finger. As a small globule of blood began to form, I used my other hand to uncover the offending object. It was a small hinged metal box, not unlike an Altoids tin, a travel-size doctor's kit from around 1900. I opened it to reveal, to my horror, the jagged remnants of broken glass vials of scary substances like strychnine and morphine. It also had a needle—previously covered in God-knows-what from God-knows-when—that had come loose and stabbed me. I sat in my sad basement office, watching my life flash before my eyes. "Is this seriously how I go out?" I wondered, as I breathed purposefully to stave off hyperventilation. I survived having learned a valuable life lesson: never stick your hand somewhere you can't see.

So there I was at Countway, trying to free this mystery object from its envelope without digging for it blindly. Eventually the contents landed in my palm. The specimen had come apart from its cardboard backing; a centuries-old, tanned piece of skin was now touching my own. Inked into it was a tattoo depicting Jesus on the cross surrounded by other people. The follicles were prominent and it was brittle like a stale cracker.

The back of the skin revealed brown swirls—as if Vincent van Gogh had gone through a scatological period—probably from glue that once held it to its cardboard backing. Now, I revel in my privilege to see amazing rare objects, to touch and smell history firsthand. But make no mistake: sometimes this work is creepy. I have a higher threshold for this stuff than a lot of people, but I am not immune.

I placed the tattooed skin back in its envelope and handed it back to the librarian. "Well, that was gross, even for me."

"Do I want to see it?" the librarian asked, and we simultaneously shook our heads. "Just a few more things were pulled for you . . . Oh, more human skin!" She feigned excitement and produced a file folder with another white envelope inside. An accompanying paper read, "Human Skin Tanned. White man's skin tanned and also colored man's skin tanned at Mullen's Tannery, North Cambridge, in 1882." But I only saw one skin specimen. It was far thicker than the previous one and had a disturbing hole. Later I would realize that hole was probably a former belly button. It hadn't crossed my jet-lagged mind when I came to Cambridge that my research might put me off my lunch. My stomach churned. Eckert was right, though: they certainly were surprises.

I met up with him later to discuss the collection. Countway had a sixteenth-century copy of Ovid's *Metamorphoses*, alleged for centuries to be bound in human skin until scientific testing revealed it to be sheepskin. "The analyses done here make me think that there are probably far fewer human skin bindings than originally thought," Eckert said. He had stumbled on anthropodermic bibliopegy in the same place I had; he worked at the College of Physicians of Philadelphia before coming to Harvard. When he heard his new workplace had an alleged human skin book, he was intrigued, but as librarians have thousands of special titles in their library to manage, he didn't give the matter too much thought. He'd occasionally bring out the book to show to the curious, but as time went by he developed a hunch that it might not be real. When Harvard Library's preservation center wanted to test the Ovid along with Harvard's other two alleged human skin books, he jumped at the chance to know the truth. "Ovid's *Metamorphoses* is all about people changing into other things, so someone changing into a book, I thought, this would be ideal." Once the truth was revealed, the Countway's copy of the *Metamorphoses* suddenly made less sense as part of a medical collection; the scientific findings changed the justification for the book's place within the library.

Upon seeing the book myself, I understood how one might think it was real. Like a lot of other alleged anthropodermic books, this one was small—about the size of my mobile phone—and the leather on the outside had very visible follicles where the hair used to grow out of the skin. Inside the front cover is a red leather bookplate adorned with a golden axe but no names or mottoes. Underneath, someone had written "bound in human skin" in pencil. Who? you might ask. It could have been anyone who encountered the book over its hundreds of years of existence—a former owner, a binder, a bookseller, a librarian. A note like this was once usually enough to convince people; with no way of being tested, a shocking claim like this tended to be taken at face value. Whatever the motivation, the act of writing "bound in human skin" inside a book placed it in the realm of anthropodermic bibliopegy and rendered it an especially unusual copy. Few things increase a book's value like scarcity.

The *Metamorphoses* seemingly had one big strike against its potential authenticity as a human skin book: its age. Untested examples with the most credible supporting historical evidence date from the late eighteenth to late nineteenth centuries. This Ovid from 1597 would seem to be too old. But before books became mechanically produced in the nineteenth century, buyers either bought a text block (the stacked and fastened pages in order, but without a cover) from the printer and then took the interior to a binder, or a bookseller would take the risk of binding text blocks and offering them for sale in his shop. It wasn't until the mid-nineteenth century that books would start coming from the publisher in the standardized, completed form of a bound hardcover that we would recognize today. The old method rendered most antiquarian books unique artifacts.

These books were resold and rebound with abandon—sometimes to personalize a book for a new owner's aesthetic tastes, sometimes to put multiple works together into one volume or take them apart. Rebinding was especially popular for nineteenth-century collectors of older rare books, so even a very old book printed before the known era of anthropodermic bibliopegy could be a human skin book, if it were rebound in the nineteenth century. Flipping through Countway's copy of the *Metamorphoses*, I noticed that some of the printed marginalia on the sides of the page were cut off, a telltale sign that it had been rebound at least once.

After years of believing that the Ovid book had this unusual distinction, some of Countway's staff were disappointed to learn that the book's binding wasn't of human origin. But Eckert was glad to have an answer. He was also not a little relieved to avoid the controversy that his Houghton colleagues faced over their real human skin book, *Des destinées de l'ame*. "The latest upheavals following the Houghton book—someone wanted to inter it; I just found that insane! Where would you stop?" Eckert was accustomed to working in medical collections that housed human remains, and shared my concerns about calls for the destruction of an artifact when so much about its individual history is unknown.

In 2014, the usually sleepy blog for Harvard University's Houghton Library announced the PMF test results of their three alleged anthropodermic books, prompting dozens of comments like these: "This book should be buried as a sign of respect for the poor patient whose body was profaned by a crazy doctor!" and "The binding is a macabre disgrace from a time when the human dignity of the mentally ill and others was readily discounted. Got any vintage WWII lampshades, Harvard?" The librarians must have been alarmed by the sudden negative attention. The announcement, then titled "Caveat Lecter," began, "Good news for fans of anthropodermic bibliopegy, bibliomaniacs and cannibals alike: tests have revealed that Houghton Library's copy of Arsène Houssaye's *Des destinées de l'ame* . . . is without a doubt bound in human skin." With this post, Harvard unintentionally brought a taboo kind of rare book into the public eye. Books bound in human skin were no longer a macabre rumor mentioned by student guides on campus tours; at least one had been confirmed as scientific fact.

Those bibliomaniacs and fans of anthropodermic bibliopegy were no doubt fascinated by Harvard's findings. Along with curiosity seekers came readers shocked both by the practice and the fact that Harvard would own such nasty things. Paul Needham, a rare book librarian at Princeton, stated that not only was the tone of the blog post "shocking in its crudity" but that the only ethical thing to do, now that the book's binding was confirmed as human, was to remove the cover and bury it. He succeeded in getting Harvard to take down the offending title and first line of the blog post, but no one interred or cremated the binding. Needham, the most vociferous voice from within the rare book world for the binding's destruction, aired his thoughts on his website and various mailing lists: "Although preservation is a central responsibility of libraries and museums, it is not one isolated from wider questions of ethics. There are times when the 'good' of preservation must be weighed against other compelling responsibilities."

Needham argued that *Des destinées de l'ame* had no research value, and furthermore, that the motivations of Ludovic Bouland, who had the book bound, were practically necrophilic: "A reader of Bouland's notes accompanying his human-skin volumes cannot miss that it was significant to Bouland that he had exerted his power upon a woman. The skin of a male would not have fulfilled his psychosexual needs in the same way. Essentially, he carried out an act of post-mortem rape."

To me, this line of thinking rings as anathema to a central tenet of what we librarians believe: we are stewards of the books in our care, especially when those books contain unpopular ideas, and we must do all we can to preserve and protect them. Though I have great professional admiration for Needham as a binding and rare book expert, I could not agree with what he asserted should be the destiny of *Des destinées de l'ame*. Like Eckert, I found it a step too far to ascribe sexual motivations to Bouland without any historical documentation.

While Needham was certainly within his right to voice his disgust at the existence of the book, I did not see why that should entitle him to call for its dismantling, thereby depriving researchers (like myself) of the ability to study it in the future. Artifacts of abominable acts have research value. I wanted to have a conversation with him to hear his full arguments, but first, I wanted to learn as much about the book as I could, starting with the man who tested it.

A SUCCESSFUL CHEMIST with stints at some big pharmaceutical companies and thirty years at IBM behind him, Daniel Kirby had begun to lose his passion for the work he was doing. Then one day, in 2003, he dropped everything to take a bike ride around the world. He started off with four strangers in Los Angeles, riding through New Zealand, across China, Southeast Asia, Europe, South Africa, and finally to South America, hopping on planes whenever oceans got in the way. Covering an average of sixty-one miles per day throughout the year, Kirby had a lot of time to think over what he wanted from his life and career. When he returned, his pharmaceutical work had lost some of its luster. "I really don't want to go back to doing that analytical work where you get an answer and throw it over the wall," Kirby said. "You have no idea what it's connected to." He wanted to feel excited about science again and see the full impact that his work could make.

Kirby thought his analytical chemistry skills might be usefully applied in museum conservation; if museums knew for sure what an art piece or artifact was made from, they would know better how to restore and protect it. Using well-established techniques from the field of proteomics (the study of proteins), Kirby could analyze the proteins in a piece of art to distinguish whether a painting's egg tempera paint contained egg yolk, egg white, or a mixture of both, and whether it came from a chicken or a duck. He analyzed indigenous Alaskan objects at Harvard's Peabody Museum of Archaeology & Ethnology, and discovered that a nineteenth-century Yup'ik kayak was stitched together with caribou and made from the skin of an earless seal (Phocidae family) and not the Steller's sea lion (Otariidae family) as previously thought, thus equipping the indigenous Alaskans who continue to make these vessels with better historical information about how their ancestors created them.

He knew that this was just the beginning of the work he could do. He and his colleague Bill Lane started identifying parchment for the Harvard conservator Alan Puglia—a seventh-century Coptic codex here, a tenth-century Koran there. When Puglia asked whether this method could be used on Harvard's three suspected cases of anthropodermic bibliopegy, Daniel Kirby found himself in the business of human skin book identification.

I met Kirby at Harvard's extensive Mass Spectrometry and Proteomics Resource Laboratory, where the other researchers greeted him over the din of lab equipment. He said his goal was to teach those working in museum and library conservation labs to perform peptide mass fingerprinting tests using affordable desktop machines. "I've taught thirty to forty people to do it already," he said. The low cost of Kirby's method and its ability to be performed by nonscientists were also appealing to conservators.

Given the perks of PMF, Kirby could easily test his way through the world's alleged anthropodermic books, sorting them into piles marked "human" and "nonhuman," right? Unfortunately, it wasn't that simple. One obstacle was identifying where these books were held, and successfully convincing libraries and museums that the tests were worthwhile. It's easy to imagine why a library might be a little reticent if they received an e-mail from a random scientist asking to test samples from their most controversial collection items. I could tell his goals were pure; he wanted to undertake a previously unexplored scientific pursuit and use his expertise to help libraries and museums learn about their collections. And it occurred to me that my own expertise could be of use: I knew many of the stewards of these collections personally; I spoke their language and understood their concerns. I decided I wanted to help.

Kirby and I compared notes on locations of alleged anthropodermic books from literature searches and word of mouth. I created a private database with information about the books, including test results, data-sharing agreements with the institutions, and photos. I set up a public website where we now receive tips and testing inquiries regularly, often from surprising places. In addition to this functional work, I also wanted to restore the books' lost histories, their contexts. I needed to visit the books and dig into their provenances.

When possible, museums provide extensive information alongside exhibitions that include human remains, such as what area of the world they came from and the approximate period of death. Accompanying cultural artifacts may tie the remains to a certain tribe or religion. Meanwhile, books bound in human skin have stripped the bodies of their context, and physically and chemically transformed the raw materials of a human being into an object. The current science can't provide evidence that would support returning books to a given cultural group or family. Even viable DNA testing couldn't tell us the race of the person who contributed to an individual binding; despite common perceptions deriving from DNA ancestry kits, there are no genetic biological distinctions among races, which are an entirely social construct. According to the biologist Joseph L. Graves, "The modern consensus of evolutionary biologists is that our species does not have enough genetic variability among its populations to justify either the identification of geographically based races or of evolutionarily distinct lineages." DNA ancestry tests merely estimate the evolutionarily recent continental origin of some segments of an individual's DNA.

To learn about the people whose bodies make up these books, we must rely on the stories that accompany the objects through the decades, allowing for the generational game of telephone that plays out as stories change to suit the times in which they are told, or disappear altogether. There is no way to change how these people were treated in their deaths, but I can restore some respect to their humanity by uncovering their stories, separating the myths from the facts, and exploring the contexts in which such treatment of the dead could be remotely acceptable.

During the early stages of our collaboration, other schools who heard about Harvard's results contacted Kirby about testing their alleged anthropodermic books. Juniata College in Pennsylvania submitted a book full of seventeenth-century law tracts called *Bibliotheca politica*, which was proven by PMF to be sheepskin. A chemist there named Richard Hark was intrigued by the process and results. He decided he wanted to work with Kirby as well. Then Kirby communicated with the Mütter Museum of the College of Physicians of Philadelphia's curator Anna Dhody, who was eager to test those alleged human skin objects I had encountered in the glass case years before. Kirby's PMF results confirmed that all five books were real human skin. This gives the Historical Medical Library of the College of Physicians of Philadelphia the bizarre distinction (among many others that they no doubt hold) of being home to the largest confirmed collection of anthropodermic books in the world.*

As the test results roll in, the Anthropodermic Book Project has established that from the known alleged cases, the number of true anthropodermic bibliopegy examples have just slightly edged out the fakes. The most prevalent commonality among these diverse human skin books is that, when the binding was created, there was almost always a doctor wielding the knife. I decided that to understand these books' real history, I needed to start at the beginning of their rumored existence and the inception of clinical medicine itself.

---

* The alleged human skin wallet that I saw on display in 2008 at the Mütter was of animal origin. Kirby also tested a number of stray skin patches—the kind of things you find lying around only at the Mütter Museum—and confirmed most to be real human skin and one to be of either elephant or mastodon origin.

{ 2 }

This Dreadful Workshop

California Rare Book School is as nerdy as it sounds, which is why I couldn't wait to go. Just two years into my librarian career and long before I visited Harvard, I was thrilled to spend a whole week in the rare book cataloging course at the University of California, Berkeley's Bancroft Library, teasing the secrets out of ancient books with monkish attention. Every day my four classmates and I were presented with cradles full of leather-bound, tooled treasures to investigate, counting the sheets of paper that had been folded and cut into gatherings called signatures, making note of disordered or missing pages, and discovering scribbles in the margins from readers hundreds of years dead. The pages—more rag than wood pulp in those days—made a glorious sound when we turned them, like boat sails bracing against the wind.

We held each page up to the light to reveal more secrets: white apparitions of lions, crowns, and other insignia that were the watermarks of papermakers. We used their position on the

page and the direction of accompanying faint white lines left
by the chains on the papermaking frame to conclude whether
the pages were folded just once (folio), twice (quarto), or more
times before they were cut and bound into the books in our
hands.

While we worked with these materials, our professor, Bancroft's head of cataloging, Randal Brandt, indulged our chatter.
We shared the dream books that we wished our institutions
owned (like I said: nerdy). I was the only medical librarian
there, so the visions of Kelmscott Chaucers dancing in my
classmates' heads, however lovely, just didn't fit into my version
of a fantasy shopping spree. My thoughts drifted back to those
strange little leather books, covers closed, that I had encountered at the Mütter Museum of the College of Physicians of
Philadelphia. Given their peculiar pedigree, they would make
for memorable props in teaching medical students about the
history and ethics at the center of their profession. With trepidation and a fear of alienating myself from our small cohort, I
mentioned these books. There was a quiet moment, and Brandt
lifted his head from his work and said thoughtfully, "Hm. I
think we have one of those."

Brandt can be forgiven for not being sure. Bancroft Library's
five-story building full of primarily special collections includes
the offices of the Mark Twain Project (the main repository of
thousands of writings by and about the iconic American hu-
morist) and an entire center devoted to the largest papyrus collection in the United States. On tours of the facility, the rows of
rare books stacks appear endless.

Thanks to a not-quite-legal parking job and the subsequent
towing, I was late to class the next morning. I burst through
the doors, sweaty and embarrassed; it was not easy to sidle in

unseen with only a half dozen people in the quiet room. The books were out on their cradles and the other students were already working. On my cradle sat a pocket-size book with a fairly modern-looking, black pebbled cover. Only the hint of a patina on the ornate silver clasps suggested its age.

Brandt gestured at the book as I was picking it up. "So I found that skin book for you," he said.

"I'm holding human leather in my bare hands," I thought to myself. "Don't freak out. Don't freak out." Funny how accustomed to it I would one day become.

I was staring down at *L'office de l'église en François* [sic], a little prayer book in Latin and French. The text block appeared well-worn but the binding was not, implying that the binding was put on some time after the 1671 printing of the text. Inside the book were two inscriptions, in pencil and in English. The first was "Bound in Human Skin." The second: "It is a matter of fact that during the horrors of the French revolution tanneries were established in various parts of France where the skins of the victims of the guillotine were tanned and some of these were used to bind books on account of the fine-grained surface exhibited after being curried. This is one of these books."

I was confused. At the time I was still under the impression that only a handful of nineteenth-century doctors had made these macabre objects, and that the College of Physicians of Philadelphia contained exceptional examples of this bizarre practice. Here I held one from a completely different time period and country, purportedly made for political reasons. I formed a mental picture of the clergyman or aristocrat who owned this book, executed by the sans-culottes. Was the holy book I held in my hands bound in human skin, perhaps that of its former owner, who was deemed an enemy of the state? If so, this was the most profane object I had ever encountered. As a new librarian enamored with the magical physicality of antique books, I was hooked. I would come to discover that the Berkeley book was far from the only French Revolution–era book carrying this eye-popping accusation.

ALONGSIDE THE INCREDIBLE but true accounts of the French Revolution's mass death and destruction, falsehoods spread like the fires set by torch-wielding mobs throughout the villages of France. Everything anyone knew under the monarchy was being challenged and dismantled. Not only were the social structures of artisan guilds, universities, and the aristocracy stripped of their authority, their physical structures were gutted and repurposed as well.

On a hill overlooking Paris from the southwest, the Château de Meudon (once a resplendent hunting lodge for Louis XV and Louis XVI after him) was ransacked by the new regime to be used for revolutionary aims. The nature of those aims has been debated for centuries. As the bodies of the executed piled high throughout France, stories propagated about Republican generals sporting culottes made of human skin as they rode into battle, and a cemetery ball where the guests were gifted human-skin-bound copies of *The Rights of Man*. If the revolutionaries actually wanted to create that many objects from human skin, artisan tanners would not be up to the task; they would have needed something more akin to a factory to meet their demands. Luckily for them, the country was newly industrializing. That factory was allegedly housed in the castle at Meudon.

The Abbot of Montgaillard is often cited as the source of the Meudon tannery rumors. Abbot Guillaume Honoré Rocques de Montgaillard worked on an epic multivolume history of France up until his death in 1825; his son Jean Gabriel Maurice Rocques, Count of Montgaillard, finished the work and published it in 1827. On a page detailing wartime technological advances, the history mentions that a new method of tanning was discovered that could fashion in just a few days leather that previously took years of preparation. An accompanying footnote translates as, "People tanned, at Meudon, human skin, and out of this dreadful workshop came the most perfectly prepared skins; the Duke of Orléans, [Philippe] Égalité, had human skin pants. The good and beautiful corpses of the tortured were skinned, and their skin tanned with particular care." The footnote goes on to note the high quality of man leather, but that women's skin wasn't as strong because of its softness. Whether this footnote was from the abbot or added by his son is unknown, but it should be noted that the Count of Montgaillard shared his father's monarchist zeal and was a secret agent on the royalist side during the Revolution and beyond. The entry in the 1911 *Encyclopædia Britannica* warns that the count's subsequent memoirs "must be read with the utmost caution."

Some moderate newspapers balked at scandalous accusations like these, but the rumors persisted. Even today, the alleged human skin tannery at Meudon is stated as fact in most writing about the practice of human skin bookbinding and in other historical accounts. "Few histories of the Revolution omit references to the infamous Royalist propaganda to the effect that a gigantic human skin tannery at Meudon filled all the requisitions for the leather goods needed by the revolutionary army quartermasters," wrote the librarian Lawrence S. Thompson, a prescient mid-twentieth-century skeptic in this historical debate.

So what was *really* going on at Meudon? There were secret machinations to be sure, but more of the standard military variety. We know that under the guidance of the engineering genius Nicolas-Jacques Conté, the Committee of Public Health converted the château's ample gardens into shooting ranges where they conducted ballistics testing of various kinds. They also explored using the new technology of hot air balloons for military purposes. When the National Convention was replaced in 1795 with a new five-person government called the Directory, one of the last acts of the Committee of Public Health was to clear out all of the workshops from Meudon, allowing only the *école d'aérostation* (the section experimenting with hot air balloons) to remain.

Into the twentieth century, the most credible chroniclers of this era's skin book rumors began to cast aspersions on the more outlandish claims of the Meudon tannery, graveyard dances, and flesh culottes. Many of them still argued that the practice did occur during the Revolution, pointing to one book as the most likely genuine article: a copy of the Constitution of 1793. The book is stored at the Musée Carnavalet in Paris, a museum dedicated to telling the story of the city through its art and cultural artifacts from the Renaissance onward. Perhaps the book's detailed provenance made it seem credible to those writing about skin books before they could be tested, but only a test can confirm or deny the claim.

I went to visit the Constitution in the two Parisian Renaissance-era townhouses whose combined grounds now serve as the Musée Carnavalet. The staff huddled with me around a small wooden table to inspect the polished mahogany book, thin and smaller than an average paperback today, with some gold-tooling and beautiful, brightly colored bubbles of marbling on the endpapers. The Constitution looked very different from the French Revolution–era book at Berkeley, but in this area of inquiry, even more than most, looks can be so deceiving.

The first few unprinted pages inside were full of handwriting that documented the march toward the new Constitution's ratification. On one page, among other bibliographic information, a note reported that the book itself was "relié en peau humaine"—"bound in human skin"; such a note, as seen with *L'office de l'église en François* and the supposed Luke Swetland parchment, is often the only indication of a potential anthropodermic book. The museum's acquisitions register made mention of this "famous binding" that "passes for human skin in imitation of calf."

The register also reported that the book once belonged to the naval officer Pierre-Charles de Villeneuve, who continued in the navy during the Revolution despite his aristocratic pedigree, until his background was discovered and he lost his captaincy in 1793. He was reinstated in 1795 after the change in power and eventually achieved the rank of vice admiral. He served under Napoleon. Repeated failures, and imprisonment by the enemy, eventually led to his suicide in 1806. After his death, the diplomat Louis Félix Étienne, marquis de Turgot, bought the book. When Étienne died in 1866, it came to the museum.

Of all the alleged anthropodermic books with a French Revolutionary provenance, this one strikes me as the most likely to be real. But that's only baseless intuition until the

book is tested. That era was unfathomably bloody and un-
moored, for sure, but was it so unruly that human skin bookbinding could thrive in the chaos?

The French Revolution sparked concomitant revolutions,
including in libraries. The Bibliothèque royale, transformed into
the newly public Bibliothèque nationale, saw its collections
swell with the contents of libraries confiscated from aristo-
crats, clergy, and conquered foreign countries. Old books were
increasingly viewed as fashionable objects worth collecting because of their physical attributes and not just their content. The
Bibliothèque nationale began amassing as many incunabula
(the earliest printed books) as possible, sparking interest in the
collection of books solely because of their age and method of
production, and regardless of the subject of the text. This shift
in the value of the physicality of the book would have lasting
repercussions on both public and private library collections.

The world of medical practice experienced its own revolutionary upheaval. In 1790, a surgeon named Cantin spoke to
the National Assembly about medical education in France, and
his beliefs would have a worldwide impact on the profession's
future: "In denouncing the past, we want to forget it; we want
to reform the present and ensure a better order for the future.
We want, in a word, that the terrible right of life and death is
conferred on those who have earned the public trust by giving
himself up to both parties at the same time."

Cantin knew that at this unusual juncture in history, everything about the structure of the French state was up for debate. The university faculties had been disbanded, opening up
questions about not just who could get an education but who
could administer one. Were degrees even necessary? Cantin
trod lightly with the crowd of revolutionaries. Abolishing the

guilds so that anyone could practice a trade was laudably egali-
tarian, Cantin argued, but in medicine, they needed *more* required education and state regulation, not less. "I will admit
that our old political bodies were contrary to liberty; but this
vice was due to their power and organization," Cantin said. He
then laid out his plan to make health care available to everyone
in the country, with legions of well-trained and government-
vetted doctors heeding the call.

To begin, doctors and surgeons would no longer belong to
two separate professions with separate standards of practice.
Before the Revolution, surgeons were regarded as holding the
same status as barbers, but afterward they were elevated to
practitioners of medicine, with all the responsibilities that des-
ignation entailed. This shift would not happen until well into
the nineteenth century in other countries. Cantin argued that
quackery, already a major problem in France when the Revolution began, would worsen if there was no state oversight of the
medical profession. "If, under the pretext of total liberty, we
permit all those who consider themselves doctors to perform
their duties, it would be authorizing impudent and ignorant
people to be nothing more than unpunished murderers . . . It
would be much better to forbid the practice of medicine altogether. At least then these daily massacres, which grow because of the decline of the art, and the respect of those who
exercise it, would be avoided." There should be a government-
licensure board for practicing physicians, and future doctors
should be trained according to a rigorous and uniform set of
standards. Apprenticeship was not enough—a doctor needed
at least three years of formal schooling, with a foundation in
subjects like anatomy and chemistry.

The rich would likely still be treated in the comfort of

their homes, but state-run hospitals—once the main purview of church charities—would bring health care to the masses by tending to the sick poor, and doctors-in-training would learn at the patients' bedsides. Medical students would also learn at the foot of the cadaver, scalpel in hand, not only identifying anatomical structures but diagnosing disease posthumously by looking at tissues and organs, a discipline known as anatomical pathology. The Parisian hospitals full of the indigent sick provided an unprecedented number of dead bodies for doctors to study.

Some of these developments in medical practice were already beginning in other European countries, but the shake-up caused by the Revolution paved the way for many radical changes to occur at once. This combination of educational requirements, pathological cadaver study, and hospital training with live patients became known worldwide as the Paris School. It would take years for some of Cantin's recommendations to be instituted fully, but the Paris School concept became the foundation for modern clinical medicine. A profound and sudden change in the way medicine was taught, it still informs the Western medical education system hundreds of years later.

In *The Birth of the Clinic*, the philosopher and social theorist Michel Foucault described how this revolutionary change in education altered the doctor-patient relationship: "The presence of disease in the body, with its tensions and its burnings, the silent world of the entrails, the whole dark underside of the body lined with endless unseeing dreams, are challenged as to their objectivity by the reductive discourse of the doctor, as well as established as multiple objects meeting his positive gaze." Foucault asserted that this style of medical education brought with it a distanced view of patients, which he referred to as the clinical gaze.

Before clinical medicine, doctors had little to go on in diagnosis besides a patient's complaints and the outward manifestations of the alleged disease on the living body. Primarily working with the wealthy, these doctors saw few patients and had widely divergent levels of training. They also didn't interact as frequently with one another as they do today, nor was there the constant continuing education now required. Their viewpoints were rather limited. The Paris School brought a scientific structure to the art of medicine and created a foundation for shared medical knowledge. It also encouraged systematic ways of learning about the body and diseases, including cadaver exploration and the use of instruments to allow doctors to observe patients' bodies in ways the patients themselves could not. The human body became a less mysterious landscape, and the patient, too, was transformed into an object to be studied—consisting of organs and the diseases that attack them.

Along the way, the medical profession lost sight of the patient as a person in favor of the patient as a collection of symptoms and manifestations, or a soulless cadaver on a dissecting table. Foucault pointed out the inherent tension between hospitals' servicing the sick and educating the doctors. He argued that, in fact, we all benefit from the advances resulting from a grossly unequal exchange:

> But to look in order to know, to show in order to teach, is not this a tacit form of violence, all the more abusive for its silence, upon a sick body that demands to be comforted, not

displayed? Can pain be a spectacle? Not only can it be, but it must be, by virtue of a subtle right that resides in the fact that no one is alone, the poor man less so than others, since he can obtain assistance only through the mediation of the rich. Since disease can be cured only if others intervene with their knowledge, their resources, their pity, since a patient can be cured only in society, it is just that the illnesses of some should be transformed into the experience of others.

The rich invest in hospitals; the poor get treated; the knowledge gained by the doctors through observation of the poor can be used to better treat the rich. The clinical gaze extended to the way the collective body of the sick was viewed as a commodity.

A few months after my trip to Paris to see the Constitution, the Bancroft Library at UC Berkeley sent samples from the profane prayer book—the one that started me wondering about French Revolution–era anthropodermic books in the first place—to Daniel Kirby for PMF testing. The results showed that the leather binding was horse. Horse! Since then, any books we've tested with an alleged French Revolution pedigree have all turned out to be made from nonhuman animals.

I would feel more comfortable concluding that the practice didn't exist at this time and place if the Constitution of 1793 were tested, though that day may never come: the Musée Carnavalet has been closed for renovations for years now, and testing their alleged anthropodermic book may not be their top priority when they open. But hope springs eternal. Regardless of whether a human skin book from this era is ever revealed, our modern system of clinical medicine surfaced from the bloody French Revolution at the same time as the rumors of anthropodermic bibliopegy, and the two practices were entwined ever after. Combined with a new upswing in the collection of books based on their physical attributes, the stage was set for an environment in which true anthropodermic bibliopegy would eventually thrive.

{ 3 }

GENTLEMEN COLLECTORS

In the summer of 1868, a twenty-eight-year-old Irish widow named Mary Lynch was admitted to Ward 27 of Philadelphia General Hospital. Nicknamed Old Blockley, this huge facility for the poor in West Philadelphia contained a hospital, an orphanage, a poorhouse, and an insane asylum. Just four summers prior, some walls in its Female Lunatic Asylum— "being undermined by workmen"—collapsed, killing eighteen women and injuring twenty more. Patient care at Blockley was a far cry from physician house calls for the wealthy; it was a place for the desperately ill poor, and Lynch's tuberculosis (then called phthisis) put her in a dire situation.

Lynch's family did what they could to make her comfortable while she suffered, visiting her with ham and bologna sandwiches in tow. No one seemed to notice the white specks on the lunchmeat—a telltale sign of roundworm infection. The trichinosis she contracted from those sandwiches compromised her already weakened state.

Nurses attended to Mary Lynch over six months as her body withered away to a mere sixty pounds. Eventually she succumbed to the two diseases wreaking havoc on her frail frame. When the young doctor John Stockton Hough first encountered Lynch, it was on his autopsy table in January 1869. In an article in *The American Journal of the Medical Sciences*, "Two Cases of Trichiniasis at the Philadelphia Hospital, Blockley," Dr. Hough reported that when he opened her chest cavity to observe her tuberculosis-ravaged lungs, he noticed that the pectoral muscles that he had sliced along the way had some unusual lemon-shaped cysts. Looking into his microscope, he realized that the cysts were teeming with *Trichinae spiralis* (worms) in various stages of development.

"Counting the number in one grain of muscle, the whole number of cysts were estimated to be about 8,000,000," Hough reported, making Lynch's the first case of trichinosis discovered in his hospital and—as far as he could find—in Philadelphia as well. It was during that autopsy that Hough removed the skin from Lynch's thighs. He preserved her skin in a chamber pot and stored it for safekeeping while the rest of Mary Lynch's body was dumped into a pauper's grave at Old Blockley.

Decades later, Dr. Hough—by then a rich, well-respected bibliophile—used Lynch's skin to bind three of his favorite medical books on women's health and reproduction, including Louis Barles's *Les nouvelles découvertes sur toutes les parties principales de l'homme, et de la femme* (1680), *Recueil des secrets de Louyse Bourgeois* (1650), and Robert Couper's *Speculations on the Mode and Appearances of Impregnation in the Human Female* (1789). Hough had cultivated a specialty in women's health beginning in his residency at Old Blockley, where he developed a speculum adaptable for vaginal, uterine, and anal use.

Dr. John Stockton Hough, like many gentlemen doctors of his day, enjoyed a classical education at the finest academies New Jersey had to offer before pursuing simultaneous degrees in chemistry and medicine at the University of Pennsylvania. During his residency at the Philadelphia General Hospital, he cultivated disparate clinical interests in reproductive medicine and parasitic *trichinae*. His family wealth and a lucrative private practice afforded him gentlemanly pursuits, and he began collecting rare books with vigor, particularly medical books from the dawn of the age of print. He traveled to Europe often, sending ahead to antiquarian booksellers a printed list of the medical incunabula he wanted to find; bibliophiles call these wish lists "desiderata." He was invited to join book collector societies like the Grolier Club in New York, established in 1884 to "foster the study, collecting, and appreciation of books and works on paper, their art, history, production, and commerce." He delighted in showing off his collection in his luxurious home library in Ewing, New Jersey, to reporters, fellow bookmen, and (on Sundays only) his own children. With a roaring fire flickering off a bookshelf stuffed with rich leather bindings, he would pull down book after book, pointing out one "nugget," "marvelous gem," or "beauty" after another.

By the time Hough was fifty, he had amassed a collection that was the envy of his fellow doctor bibliophiles; he estimated in 1880 that he owned around eight thousand books. His copy of Fabricius ab Acquapendente's *De formato foetu* (1627) was rare to start, but Hough's copy was made unique by its thirty painted folios illustrating fetal development. He also had a few examples of anatomical texts from the late sixteenth and early seventeenth centuries that featured anatomical flap illustrations, reminiscent of today's children's books, where flap after flap lifts to reveal the layers of body structures doctors would encounter as they dissected a cadaver. Few of these books survive today given the centuries of curious fingers folding their flaps. Hidden among these gems, looking much the same as any other book on the shelf, were the three works on reproduction bound in the skin of Mary Lynch. Hough died at age fifty-six after a runaway horse threw him from his carriage, and the bulk of his prized collection went to Hough's alma mater, the University of Pennsylvania, and the library at the College of Physicians of Philadelphia.

While the identities of most of the patients used by doctors to create human skin books are lost to history, the doctors who created them were often well respected in their fields, admired doctors and collectors occupying elevated social strata in a nineteenth-century United States clamoring for the legitimacy of its European counterparts. Unlike most doctors who created these books, Hough gave some identifying information about the source of his leather in his handwritten notes inside, referring to "Mary L___" in each of the three volumes made from her skin. It was this tidbit, plus her knowledge of Hough's tenure at Old Blockley, that inspired the College of Physicians of Philadelphia librarian Beth Lander to dig into the Philadelphia General Hospital archives in search of the true identity of the woman who supplied the skin for three out of their five confirmed anthropodermic books.

"THIS BOOK IS THE BIGGEST PAIN," sighed John Pollack, a rare book librarian at the University of Pennsylvania. In my travels studying anthropodermic bibliopegy, I would soon become accustomed to this reaction from my fellow librarians. "A research library full of amazing stuff and people want to see this," he said as he hefted the massive book in his hands.

I try to hedge a little about the types of titles that tend to be bound in human skin, as it takes only one confirmation of a certain kind of book to completely change our understanding of the universe of this practice. People often ask me if there are "sexy" human skin books, and I used to say no—until we tested a nineteenth-century printing of a sixteenth-century French BDSM allegorical poem, owned by that same Grolier Club to which Hough belonged, and lo and behold: real human skin. Even so, I have come to see certain traits that tip the scale toward whether an untested book might be real or fake.

To my eye, then, this doorstop at Penn had fake written all over it. It was Hough's copy of the *Catalog des sciences médicales* (Catalog of Medical Sciences) from the Bibliothèque nationale de France. It contains lists of medical works housed at the library in that era, like a nineteenth-century library's equivalent of a phone directory. It's quarter-bound, meaning only one quarter of the book is covered in leather, around the spine, and the front and back covers of the book are more like what we would recognize as a hardcover today, with paper over board. It is so big that opening and closing over the years has put a lot of strain on the binding, which has developed red rot, an irreversible condition in which exposure to acids begins to break down the leather. The library covered it in a clear mylar jacket to stop the red rot from depositing bits of putative human leather on anyone who handles the book.

The real human skin books that our scientific team has verified over the years have content that was specifically chosen to match their macabre binding. The books that Hough bound in Mary Lynch's skin were about women's medicine, bound in the skin of a woman whose hide he held on to for decades before using it. So why would that same person use the world's rarest binding material to bind a *directory*? Pollack, too, was incredulous: "I feel like he picked the most boring book off his shelf and said, 'Oh, this will do.'" This book will always remind me not to lean too heavily on my initial instincts, because a few months prior to my visit, Penn had sent a sample to Daniel Kirby, and the testing results confirmed the binding of *Catalog des sciences médicales* as real human skin.

I might never know the full story behind this misfit skin book, but I slowly started connecting the dots to form a more complete picture of Hough as a gentleman collector. Hough was a bibliographer who loved compiling lists of desiderata, and he also attempted to quantify the world's rarest medical books in lists. Inside the *Catalog* he wrote, "The Bibliotheque National [*sic*] in 1889 contained 15,000 incunabula of all kinds, of which a catalogue is being prepared, if 1 out of 30 books are medical there would be 500 medical books printed in the XV Century." That kind of listmaking might sound boring to me and John Pollack, but it must have been pretty exciting to Hough, as he was attempting to define the universe of medical incunabula and collect as many as possible—not unlike the Bibliothèque nationale's own tactics in the wake of the French Revolution. Above that note was another that read, "Bound with skin from the back-tanned June 1887," and directly below that, "bound Jany. 1888." But there is also a note on that same page that reads "Stockton-Hough, Paris, Sept. 1887." It is possible he went back to this page multiple times to update these notes.

The notes in the *Catalog* reveal that the skin was tanned and the book bound in quick succession, without the intervening decades of storage like the other Hough anthropodermic books, which leads me to wonder whether the inveterate bibliophile, having finally run out of saved skins to bind books, procured more skin to try his hand at binding books himself. The *Catalog* lacks the gilded embellishments and other signs of skilled craftsmanship of the other specimens that he had created. Those specimens all appear to have been made by the same craftsman. The red rot now affecting the book could be a side effect of some of the newer tannins being used at the time, or it could have been made by someone with less expertise. Perhaps the *Catalog* was the result of Hough's attempt at bookbinding—perhaps he truly did, as Pollack joked, pull any old book off the shelf and say, "This'll do."

The College of Physicians of Philadelphia owns a fourth anthropodermic book, also about reproduction, from John Stockton Hough's collection: Charles Drelincourt's *De conceptione adversaria* (1686). On the flyleaf inside, Hough's handwritten note reveals that it was bound in Trenton, New Jersey, in March 1887, using the "skin from around the wrist of a man who died in the [Philadelphia] Hospital 1869—Tanned by J.S.H. 1869. This bit of leather never boiled or curried." To curry, in this case, means dressing the already tanned hides by soaking, scraping, or dyeing to achieve a certain look and feel.

I returned to Hough's article on the two cases of trichinosis. Mary Lynch was the first. The other is described as an "intemperate" forty-two-year-old Irish laborer he called "T McC," who died in February 1869, emaciated and having suffered from chronic diarrhea (just like Mary Lynch). Hough found *Trichinae spiralis* during his autopsy as well. Could he be the man whose wrist supplied the binding for the Drelincourt book?

A dig through the Philadelphia General Hospital's Male Register turned up a Thomas McCloskey whose intake and discharge dates all align with those reported by Hough in his article. The timing certainly matches, but since Hough merely describes him, on the book's flyleaf, as "a man who died in the [Philadelphia] Hospital 1869," I can't draw as bright a line there as Beth Lander could between Mary Lynch's hospital records and the "Mary L___" in Hough's handwriting.

If your mental image of a doctor binding books in human skin is that of a lone mad scientist, toiling away in a creepy basement creating abominations, that would be understandable. But the truth about these doctors is much harder to square with our current perceptions of medical ethics, consent, and the use of human remains. Meanwhile, Hough wasn't even the only one in Philadelphia at that time making human skin books.

When Mary Lynch was ailing in Old Blockley in 1868, there was a doctor and illustrious scientist working in Philadelphia who would have cautioned her to throw away her wormy sandwiches, potentially saving her life. But Joseph Leidy's discovery that *Trichinae spiralis* in pork was the cause of trichinosis in humans, and his warnings to thoroughly cook pork to avoid contracting the disease, went unrecognized by the medical community for decades. Even if his colleagues had listened to him, word would probably never have reached the likes of Lynch's family. Despite the small footprint of the city of Philadelphia, Leidy and Lynch occupied two completely distinct worlds. Leidy's Philadelphia was that of a striving middle class, with countless professional and hobby societies full of scientific dilettantes and gentlemen collectors. Philadelphia for Lynch meant overcrowded, polluted slums experiencing rapid industrialization, and if you caught one of the diseases like tuberculosis that raged through the city, your fate was all but sealed.

ABOUT TWENTY YEARS before the death of Mary Lynch, Leidy was poking at his breakfast ham with a fork when he noticed some white specks in the meat. He promptly examined his meal with a microscope. In the 1840s, the microscope was seldom employed in clinical medicine but was sometimes used for botanical or zoological study. Leidy received his first microscope as a childhood present from his mother; he delighted in losing himself in the world of microbes, and often gifted microscopes to his friends. He was a shy boy with a strong curiosity about the natural world and a talent for drawing what he found in nature. But while Leidy's passion lay in science (then viewed mostly as a hobby, not a practical career), his mother insisted he apply himself to the practice of medicine to attain the elevated class comforts that the profession provided.

At the time that Leidy began studying medicine in the 1840s, Americans were just beginning to make their mark in the European-dominated profession. Yet in 1847, the first president of the American Medical Association, Nathaniel Chapman, was already mourning the bygone era of colonial medicine as preferable to the jockeying for social standing he saw in his fellow Philadelphia doctors: "The profession to which we belong, once venerated on account of its antiquity—its varied and profound science—its elegant literature—its polite accomplishments—its virtues—has become corrupt and degenerate, to the forfeiture of its social position, and with it, of the homage it formerly received spontaneously and universally." Later, one of Chapman and Leidy's University of Pennsylvania colleagues would beg to differ. William Osler—another microscope enthusiast, the father of modern American clinical medicine, and one of the greatest medical book collectors—viewed doctors as representatives of a certain class of gentlemen, belonging to many social clubs, collecting finer things, and serving as exemplars of their communities. A doctor who didn't read avidly was unthinkable to Osler:

> For the general practitioner a well-used library is one of the few correctives of the premature senility which is so apt to overtake him. Self-centered, self-taught, he leads a solitary life, and unless his every-day experience is controlled by careful reading or by the attrition of a medical society it soon ceases to be of the slightest value and becomes a mere accretion of isolated facts, without correlation. It is astonishing with how little reading a doctor can practice medicine, but it is not astonishing how badly he may do it.

Osler even praised bibliomaniacs, a tongue-in-cheek diagnosis given to the learned book collectors who were so obsessive in their acquisitions that the contents of the book often didn't matter as much as the beauty and scarcity of the object itself. "We need more men of their class," Osler proclaimed to a crowd of fellow doctor bibliophiles at the opening of the Boston Medical Library in 1901, "particularly in this country, where every one [sic] carries in his pocket the tape-measure of utility."

Just when clinical detachment was becoming more cemented in medical practice, doctors were getting social cues from their leaders about the importance of object acquisition. Over the course of the latter half of the nineteenth century, leisure pursuits such as rare book collecting would become deeply ingrained in what it meant to be a member of the doctoring class in America.

For his part, the young Joseph Leidy did not seem concerned with putting on gentlemanly airs. His colleagues described him as "devoid of personal ambition," a person who seemed "to have sought positions not for the distinction they might bring to him, but only for the opportunity which they might afford for the pursuit of his scientific studies." His relatives remembered that his "gentle, sympathetic and emotional nature was such that he could not witness pain or suffering in man or beast. These characteristics never diminished but increased with advancing years." According to his biographer Leonard Warren, "Quite simply, there were no skeletons in the closet of this enigmatic man."

Despite his scientific talents, Leidy never really grew comfortable as a practitioner of medicine. As a teen, he observed dissections at the Philadelphia School of Anatomy and "was so disgusted with the dissecting room," he recalled, "that after spending the first half day there, I went away and could not be induced to return for six weeks and did not get over the melancholy of it for a year." Eventually he summoned the courage to return and soon became quite skilled at dissections, impressing far more experienced anatomists with his ability to isolate obscure anatomical structures.

While his comfort with the dead body improved, living patients stymied Leidy. Legend has it that when his first patient approached the gate of his Philadelphia home office, Leidy panicked, locked the door, and hid. Leidy was not unaware that his bedside manner was lacking, and he abandoned private practice as soon as he could. He distinguished himself as a leader in the burgeoning field of paleontology instead, and continued dissecting dead humans to make a living as an anatomical prosector. Not only was he sought after as a dissector and later professor, but he also worked for the Philadelphia coroner's office, putting his skills to use on some of the city's earliest crimes solved by forensic means. Armed with his microscope and scalpel, Leidy worked with the human body from a new, minute, and abstracted vantage point.

Despite his early misgivings, Leidy was soon right at home in the anatomy lab. Back in the 1850s, anyone entering the University of Pennsylvania's medical building on Ninth Street might have been lucky enough to pass Leidy's colleague Fred Schafhirt dissecting reptiles while drinking schnapps and jauntily singing German patriotic songs. The mood likely changed considerably if this passerby walked to the adjoining room where the reserved Leidy performed dissections alongside his lay assistant, Bob Nash. Leidy had treated Nash for a broken thigh at the hospital and—thinking his bulk and strength could be of use in the anatomy lab—hired him thereafter. A loyal guardian at Leidy's gate and a skilled dissector in his own right, Nash kept the rougher elements away and helped fill the requests for anatomical specimen preparations that Leidy received from around the world.

On the same floor, Leidy curated an anatomical museum that he filled with his best preparations of both normal and pathological anatomy. Leidy accomplished all of this work early on in his career; he was thirty-one years old when he addressed his first anatomy class as a professor. In that first lecture, he framed human anatomy as inherently comparative anatomy. The human body, to Leidy, deserved no more special consideration than those of animals, which was a maverick view, but one that was beginning to gain acceptance in the new age of Darwin.

To doctors of Leidy's era, the corpse was king. Dissecting corpses in the anatomy lab opened up a whole new world to the clinician, revealing the innermost secrets of the human body, with the side effect that doctors came to view these bodies as inert objects to be studied, like the seashells or feathers in a cabinet of curiosities. Leidy advocated strongly for the importance of human cadavers in medical education and was less than impressed with the practicality of the anatomy books available to teach his students alongside the dissections. His solution was to write his own book, *An Elementary Treatise on Human Anatomy* (1861). Its 663 pages featured nearly four hundred anatomical illustrations, mostly drawn by Leidy himself. Because he wanted to provide anatomy students with the most practical anatomical text to use while dissecting, he checked the proofs of the book in front of an open cadaver before sending it to be printed.

Leidy's accessible anatomical text must have been appreciated during the Civil War, when battle casualties and amputations abounded. Business at the medical school ground to a halt, with Philadelphia's large Southern student population leaving in droves to fight. Leidy's mother, a staunch abolitionist, insisted that her four sons contribute to the war effort. "If I had a dozen sons they would all go," she said. Leidy's brothers became casualties of the war, two dying in action and one succumbing to his war injuries years later. For his part, Joseph carried out volunteer scientific work for the War Department and the Sanitary Commission, and performed surgeries at Satterlee military hospital in West Philadelphia. And it was likely at the military hospital that he pocketed a slice of skin from a dead soldier.

THROUGHOUT HIS LONG CAREER, Joseph Leidy published hundreds of scientific articles, but his *Elementary Treatise* was special to him and his family. His inscription in one copy revealed that he bound it in "human skin, from a soldier who died during the great southern rebellion." When his nephew's wife donated the copy to the College of Physicians of Philadelphia, she described it as one of her husband's most prized possessions. This book rests today with John Stockton Hough's four anthropodermic books, making the College library home to the largest confirmed collection of anthropodermic books in the world. Two young doctors, working in the same city on some of the same clinical problems with the same distanced eye and collector's mindset, created this hoard of human skin books.

Leidy's contributions to the College's collections did not end there. In 1858, the College of Physicians of Philadelphia saw a need for a museum for pathological anatomy to ensure that important specimens were preserved and available to scientific study. Leidy, who was part of a worldwide network of collectors of artifacts from the natural world, took it upon himself to help the fledgling Mütter Museum acquire specimens of the rarest deformities and diseases. His acquisition methods were not ethical by today's standards.

In 1875, Leidy brought the mysterious Soap Lady to the Mütter. When he heard about some unusual bodies that had been uncovered during construction work downtown, he rushed over to purchase them—one for the Mütter and one for the Wistar Institute, then housed at the University of

Pennsylvania. In the airless subterranean environment, the fat in the corpses had chemically reacted with the soil's basic pH, preserving and transforming them into adipocere, a waxy substance similar to soap. In 1896, after Leidy's death, Dr. William Hunt, who was acting curator of the Mütter Museum in 1875, told the Philadelphia *Public Ledger* about how excited Leidy was to procure the bodies, only to be met at the construction site by the superintendent, who:

> put on airs, talked of violating graves, etc.; so the discomfited doctor was about to withdraw. Just then the Superintendent touched him significantly on the elbow and said: "I tell you what I do, I give bodies up to the order of relatives." The doctor took the hint, went home, hired a furniture wagon, and armed the driver with an order reading: "Please deliver to bearer the bodies of my grandfather and grandmother." This brought the coveted prizes and the virtuous caretaker was not forgotten.

Leidy invoiced the museum for $7.50, which he noted on the receipt as "one-half the sum paid persons through whose connivance I was able to procure two adipocere bodies." This doctor had a lot of skeletons in his closet after all.

Leidy told the Mütter that the corpse he had brought them was the body of a middle-aged or old woman named Ellenbogen, that she was a victim of the yellow fever epidemic in 1792, and that her body was recovered from an unearthed cemetery at Fourth and Race Streets. Over time, Mütter Museum curators and scientists with CT scanners would come to understand none of his claims could have been true. The woman who came to be known as the Soap Lady was probably in her twenties when she died in the early nineteenth century, during an era without a yellow fever epidemic; her name was not Ellenbogen; no cemetery ever existed at that location. Now she is enclosed in a glass case on the second floor of the museum, and modern researchers at the Mütter continue to apply new scientific techniques to the old historical questions she raises, much like the work I and my colleagues are doing with the anthropodermic books in the museum's collection.

In that way, the original educational mission of this pathological museum continues to bear fruit. In 2016, when construction unearthed an eighteenth-century burial ground just a few blocks from where Leidy purported to find the Soap Lady, the current curator, Anna Dhody, sprang into action, but with a very different mindset from Leidy's. Dhody and her team of volunteer forensic professionals and archaeologists uncovered 491 bodies from the forgotten cemetery and removed them from the site. They will be stored safely and eventually analyzed to gain a better picture of what life and death were like for Philadelphians at the time. In a particularly twenty-first-century twist, their Arch Street Bones Project was crowdfunded to cover the costs of this venture. In a few years, when the study is complete, the bones will be reinterred at the historic Mount Moriah Cemetery. Dhody said that the Mütter "felt like we had a moral obligation to do what we could." Same museum, similar circumstances, but the intervening 141 years completely changed the ethics of how the bodies were procured and what will be done with them once they have been studied.

On one of my visits to the Mütter, Dhody showed me a workshop filled with the bones they have uncovered and studied. I marveled that I was standing next to skulls and femurs likely put in the ground before this country was founded. I was witnessing the exciting collision of history and science first-hand, which is just how I feel about our Anthropodermic Book Project work. If it weren't for the endurance of these objects, carefully attended to by library and museum staff, we wouldn't be able to study them with today's technologies and interrogate them through our updated lenses. After a while, people could question whether these objects ever existed, eventually dismissing them as too incredible to be anything but legend.

Objects cared for in libraries and museums retain their all-important context, and new contexts are added over time, as long as the objects are permitted to persist. For example, the new display of the Soap Lady highlights the fact that Leidy used unethical means to add her to the collection, thereby teaching about the history of the liberties doctors have taken with bodies like hers. Caring for these unusual objects so that they can be studied by scholars far into the future is a tricky business in itself. It helps to know how and from what they were made, but that information is not always so easy to find. I was getting more and more curious about how Hough could have gone about transforming Mary Lynch into leather, so I went to ask one of the only people in the country who might know.

{ 4 }

SKIN CRAFT

My research trips tend to resemble the first twenty minutes of a horror movie—a woman alone, naively plunging headlong into some mystery she has no business investigating, driven by a vague curiosity and a disdain for common sense. This time I drove my rental car down Factory Street, across old train tracks overgrown with the beautiful greenery of New York's Hudson River Valley in full bloom. There was a big part of the history of these books that I still didn't understand, and I thought a field trip was in order.

John Stockton Hough noted in one of his books that he tanned Mary Lynch's skin in a chamber pot—one of the only clues I had found as to how human skin tanning was actually accomplished at the time—but I had little concept of what else Hough needed to do in order to make this patient into a book. The few bookbinders who have written in professional journals about the human leather tanning process reported that it was more or less the same as for tanning animal hides, assuming their contemporaries would understand what that meant. But finding step-by-step information on how leather was tanned in the nineteenth century—and discerning what might have been different when tanning a person's skin—was proving difficult. This kind of knowledge was usually passed from skilled artisan to apprentice and rarely written down.

I discovered that almost no one in the world still uses the historical vegetable leather tanning methods that a doctor or his hired tanner would have employed on a human skin; after the Industrial Revolution, most tanners switched to using a chromium solution that dramatically shortens the tanning process. Anthropodermic bibliopegy seemed to me to straddle a time period when the profession was moving to new, larger-scale industrial methods, but some individuals would still have had the working knowledge of the old ways to put to use for this strange purpose. Today one of the only places in the United States still tanning leather the old-fashioned way is called Pergamena, named after the ancient Greek city of Pergamon (in modern Turkey), where parchment from animal skins was developed as a replacement for papyrus for writing.

I first heard about Pergamena while chatting with a leather accessories artisan who had taken a workshop there. He said that all of the attendees had to wear tall rubber boots, and just as he was thinking that was overkill, the instructor opened a drum and a wave of effluent cascaded out. He swore that he saw actual goat testicles float by his feet. "This is going to sound weird," I said, "but I think I have to go see these goat balls for myself." So during a work trip to New York, I rented a car and drove alone into the woods.

As I sheepishly ducked my head into Pergamena tannery's open door, I looked to my left to see a pile of calf hides, their fur caked in salt and sprinkled with flies. As a former longtime vegan, I was pretty nervous about how I would handle this visit, particularly the smell of a tannery, which I had read was among the worst smells one could imagine. I was surprised, then, that these hides smelled pretty much like wet dog. "Not so bad," I thought, but as I turned my head to the right, I was hit full force in the face with the most repugnant smell I had ever encountered.

Since then I have tried in vain to describe this odor succinctly. A food writer friend had once recommended that I try a tripe sandwich made from *lampredotto* (a cow's fourth stomach) during my honeymoon in Florence. My husband, Etan, gamely ordered the sandwich while I opted for something tamer. I had never seen my husband fail to finish a meal, but two bites in, he gave up on the *lampredotto*. I tasted it and nearly vomited after the first bite. I couldn't get the taste out of my mouth for hours afterward.

That's the closest I can come to communicating the nature of the smell coming off the vat of wastewater at that tannery in July. It was not merely a smell—it felt like having raw animal organs stuffed into my mouth and pulled through my nose.

Just then, Jesse Meyer bounded down the stairs and greeted me. "I didn't know I'd have to do this part today," he said, gesturing over to some massive metal drums. "I would have worn my boots." I looked down at my own worn-out Keds. I stepped gingerly as I followed him over to the drums, but soon realized there was no avoiding the slick of ooze on the floor, which resembled Mountain Dew with chunks of fat floating in it. He tossed some hides into the drum and led me upstairs to dry land to meet his dad and brother.

PERGAMENA, ONCE CALLED Richard E. Meyer & Sons, is a family business with an unbelievably long history—prior to coming to America in 1830, the Meyers had been tanning leather in Germany since 1550. There were even Meyers tanning in the Philadelphia and New Jersey areas around the same time that Leidy, Lynch, and Hough lived there. Over the decades, the business focused mainly on supplying leather for bowling shoes and parts for Steinway pianos. As that business started to dwindle, the family thought their company might go under. By the turn of the twenty-first century, small American tanneries were in a bind. They wouldn't be able to afford to keep up with environmental regulations if they switched to the heavily polluting chrome tanning method; they couldn't compete with the chrome tanneries' output if they stuck with the more environmentally sustainable, but slower, vegetable tanning process. While massive new chrome tanneries could process 6,500 hides in a day, the Meyers' small operation churned out about 40 hides a week. Then the eldest son, Jesse, returned from art school in 1995 and started experimenting with making parchment. They slowly began providing parchment and leathers for high-end specialty uses, including for books and manuscripts. Pergamena found a new customer base.

Nowadays Jesse Meyer hosts workshops attended by rare book and manuscript conservators trying to save objects, as well as historians trying to piece together the mechanics of important crafts made by processes now lost to us. "You have a parchment-bound book, or a book of hours that has tissue-thin parchment pages that is priceless," Meyer said. Researchers can't really play around with priceless antiquities like those, but they can experiment with new materials made using the old methods, a rare opportunity that Pergamena provides. "You can figure out what its limitations are, how much it can withstand, what temperature, tear strength, where all these markings on the hide come from."

Meyer has also assisted in early biocodicology studies, for example, by supplying expertise and parchments for analysis in the development of an eraser-rubbing sample-gathering technique. This method was applied to ultrafine thirteenth-century "uterine vellum"—purported to be the skin of fetal calves—and ruled out some other rumored animals of origin for the skin, like rabbit and squirrel.

"Although the use of genuine uterine vellum cannot be discounted," wrote Sarah Fiddyment in her team's 2015 *Proceedings of the National Academy of Sciences* article, "our results suggest that its availability was not a defining factor in medieval parchment production. Instead, our findings would seem to emphasize dependence on a highly specialized craft technique rather than the supply of a particular raw material. A more likely explanation for the production of fine parchment is the use of relatively young animals and the deployment of specific finishing techniques that enabled the corium to be ground to the desired thickness." Fiddyment further suggested that these new scientific investigations of old books could give archaeologists valuable insight into historical livestock economies. Skilled artisans like Jesse Meyer help scholars bridge the gaps in our historical knowledge of every-day trades.

JESSE MEYER AND I perched on a bench in a room stocked floor to ceiling with rolls of creamy leathers in every imaginable color. There, we cobbled together the little evidence I had from Hough's notes to figure out how he and others like him might have gone about transforming a corpse on a dissecting table into a human leather-bound book. Meyer is a process geek to the highest level and has clearly done this kind of historical hashing-out with others; I was delighted to pick his brain. Hough wrote that Lynch's skin was "tanned in a 'pot de chambre' by J. S-H." If he used urine in that chamber pot to preserve the skin before tanning, he may have added salt to prevent decay. The naturally occurring acid and salt in urine would have acted as a pickling brine, which Meyer said was a common hide preservation tactic in the era to keep the skin free from bacteria, fungus, and mold until it could be tanned properly.

If Hough or someone he hired continued in the traditional tanning methods of the time, he would have washed the skin, and maybe added lime (calcium hydroxide) to remove the hair and other debris still attached to it; the ammonia created when urine sits over time (sometimes historically known as lant or chamber-lye) could also have a similar effect. The liming process could take up to a week in those days. On one hand, there probably was not much hair to remove from Lynch's thighs compared to an animal's, but on the other, human follicles are deeper than those of most animals used to make leather. This could explain why the follicles are prominent on the four

Hough books at the College of Physicians of Philadelphia (though they aren't *always* prominent on anthropodermic books). Then the preparer may have used a draw knife or some other dull blade to scrape the skin further, possibly repeating the liming and scraping process a few times until he achieved the desired look.

The next step, called bating, required digestive enzymes to remove grease and blood and make the leather larger and with a better drape. Now those enzymes come in powder form, but back then you could use any rotting matter—usually animal dung—to do the job. After another wash, it would finally be ready to tan into leather. Some other alleged anthropodermic books have notes mentioning they were tanned in sumac; other high-tannin plants such as oak, chestnut, and mimosa were also commonly used in producing what is now called vegetable-tanned or vegetan leather. Meyer said the drums in his tannery are used to complete all of these steps more quickly, because the movement helps the tannins integrate completely into the hide. Historically, each step could take weeks or months of processing in outdoor pits—longer if the leather was also dyed.

Meyer picked up some examples of finished but undyed vegetable tanned leather to show me the subtle variations produced by different tannins; most impart just a tinge of brown and sometimes pink. I have seen anthropodermic books dyed many of the same colors as animal leather-bound books of that era. He gave one a sniff. "It's a very nice smell, sweet and woody," he said as he held it under my nose. "It always reminds me a little bit of baked beans." (I was a little skeptical about Meyer's sense of smell, given that he worked in the tannery every day, but he was right; the baked beans were a vast improvement over the *lampredotto*.)

The College of Physicians of Philadelphia librarian Beth Lander suggested that perhaps Hough used urine alone to tan the skin, as people today mix urine and water to preserve fish skins. Some contemporary Native Alaskan artists have been experimenting with fish tanning in an attempt to reverse-engineer their ancestors' bags and coats, because the handed-down knowledge of the traditional processes has been lost.

Meyer said the fish "tanning" process isn't really tanning at all, but a different kind of preservation method. "Fish oils and fats might keep the skin flexible, and the process of oil tanning has been practiced for ages, where oils are added to a skin which will slowly ferment creating aldehyde compounds, which are preservatives," Meyer said. "This is a different process, though, from the tanning process normally used in making book leather, where vegetable tannins are used." Though some use the word *tanning* to describe it, technically the fish skin is still raw like parchment and the chemical reaction that renders it into leather (and therefore permanently impervious to rot, moisture, and heat) has not taken place. This distinction is why parchment pages or book covers will expand and warp under high humidity or shrink and become brittle in an environment that is too dry, while leather books are much more shelf stable, though maintaining a stable environment is best for the long-term preservation of both.

After I showed him some photos of Hough's books, he confirmed that they were clearly tanned in a more traditional vegetable tanning process like other book leathers of their day. "I don't think they were made just using urine," Meyer said. "I've never heard of this preparation method being associated with leather or book production and the time period, place, and manner of decoration all point to using conventional tanning methods of the time. Using urine to prep the skin in the chamber pot might make sense, but not all by itself."

It seemed likely that what Hough called tanning was actually just the first step of the preservation process with urine, and shortly afterward he sent it to a tanner to finish the job, or perhaps finished the tanning himself. Given Hough's tendency to make notes in his books about their dates and the processes applied to make them, I would think that if he tanned the leather himself he would have mentioned what plant he used as a tannin, for example. While there are famous bookbinders in history—some who even signed their work— leather tanners' names weren't often recorded. I suspect most doctors who made anthropodermic books took only the first step of temporarily preserving the skins—probably in urine, readily available at the hospitals where they worked—before sending them to a professional to do the rest. The resulting dried and stable leather is most likely what Hough kept for decades, not the wet, pickled skin.

Now that I had an idea of all that went into making the leather, I was more gobsmacked than ever at Hough's detachment; how removed he must have felt from the patients at Blockley, how little he must have thought of Lynch's humanity, in order to bind her into his favorite books. Even if he gave the pickled skin to someone else to tan, it was an exceedingly dirty business.

That said, after a few hours of palling around with Jesse Meyer at the tannery, I found that my comfort level with all the dead animal parts increased dramatically without my even realizing it was happening. As a responsible journalist, I felt the need to fact-check the story of the floating goat balls. Meyer laughed at the question and confirmed that, yes, that was a common enough occurrence. He told me that all of their skins come from animals slaughtered for food, and that the butchers slit the animals' throats while they're still alive to make sure the pumping of their hearts removes as much of the blood as possible; too much blood left in the body could pool, affecting the hide. He began miming how the skins are removed, stressing the importance of skinning the animal when it is freshly dead, before rigor mortis sets in. Often animals' sex organs stay with the hide when it goes to the tannery, and Jesse talked about coming across some errant testicles or a penis "that feels like a big, thick piece of rigatoni." I couldn't help but laugh at the revolting imagery. "That's what I have in that steel drum downstairs. I'm rehydrating those calf skins and now I have to go wash them and start dehairing," Meyer said, checking the time. "You're welcome to hang around and watch, but I need to go put boots on and take care of that."

I said my goodbyes, wiped my Keds in the grass outside, and hopped back into my car, happy to return to breathing fully. But the smell followed me. I drove a few blocks to a coffee shop and realized that the gummy souls of my sneakers had been saturated with that fatty Mountain Dew stuff and the stink that went with it. I would never be able to explain to the rental place how I befouled their car with this unholy funk. I took off my shoes, got out of the car, and pitched them right into the trash can. Luckily I had a spare pair of sandals with me.

On the long drive down to Philadelphia, thoughts of Dr. Hough mingled with a deepened appreciation for the material craft that went into making handmade books, the artisanal industries withering away, and the irreplaceable knowledge that disappears with it all. I also thought about the rigatoni and goat balls, and wondered: Where was the me who spent twelve years as a vegan for animal rights reasons, while current me was yukking it up in that tannery? If I could be desensitized that quickly and easily to animal gore, why was it so surprising to me that a doctor, exposed every day to the horrors of a nineteenth-century autopsy table, could lose sight of the humanity of the people on the slab?

As the voices on the radio ads changed to that familiar Philadelphia accent I grew up with, I wondered if the folks at the College of Physicians of Philadelphia were going to start getting sick of all my visits. This time, I wanted to return to the work of a woman writer more than four hundred years dead, whose book Hough chose to bind in Mary Lynch's skin.

{ 5 }

SECRETS OF THE SAGES-FEMMES

I n the fall of 1601, Louise Bourgeois Boursier found herself
at the bedside of the queen of France, Marie de Médicis,
assisting with the birth of the dauphin Louis XIII. While
the queen labored, a crush of two hundred people filled her
room and spilled out into the adjacent rooms. Furious at the
encroachment into the birthing chamber but trying to keep
her composure, Bourgeois told the king he had to dismiss the
onlookers, to which he replied, "Hush, hush, midwife, do not
be angry at all, this child belongs to everyone, everyone must
rejoice."

Despite the hectic scene, Bourgeois maintained her professionalism and delivered the dauphin successfully. She was
taking the advice that she gave midwives-in-training: "Above
all, I advise you, whatever may happen, never seem to be at
a loss; for there is nothing so unpleasant to witness as those
households all at sixes and sevens." Her approach was to intervene in the birth as little as possible, to avoid excessive manual

examinations and never to break membranes; the baby would come when he and the mother were ready. Employing this mindset, Bourgeois would go on to deliver five more of the royal couple's children.

Thanks to her stellar track record with the French royal family, Bourgeois and her midwifery skills were in high demand throughout Parisian aristocratic and bourgeois society, and she did brisk business birthing the babies of the elite. The wife of an assistant to the legendary surgeon Ambroise Paré, she learned anatomy and encouraged other midwives to do the same, cautioning, "If [the midwife] does not know this she may try to expel the uterus instead of the placenta."

Bourgeois could read Latin, and in 1609 she published the earliest midwifery manual written by a woman, called *Observations diverses sur la stérilité, perte de fruict, fécondité, accouchements et maladies des femmes*. It would be translated into Latin, German, Dutch, and English. In French, the word for midwife is *sage-femme*, which translates literally to "wise woman." Bourgeois built her reputation accordingly, but also called upon a doctor or surgeon when needed.

The top of the title page of *Observations* features an engraving of a beaming royal couple with their child. To the left of the title, a round-bellied mother holds a baby; to the right, a midwife holds a bucket and herbs. Surrounding these figures are the Latin phrases *Timor Dei* and *Gratia Dei*— "Fear God" and "Thank God." The overall impression is one of gratitude and serenity.

A competing work by the surgeon Jacques Guillemeau, entitled *De l'heureux accouchement des femmes* (roughly: On Happy Childbirth by Women), appeared the next year. The 1621 edition of this book, renamed *De la grossesse et accouchement des femmes* (On Pregnancy and Childbirth by Women—the happiness part notably removed) included a title page that featured two cherubs holding a terrifying jumble of metal clamps and forceps, like those used by surgeons attending a birth. Jacques Guillemeau's son Charles wrote the note to the reader, stating that the *sages-femmes* could learn from his father's work as well, and if they weren't so vain about their profession they would "recognize in it a number of defects as regards the skill of the deliveries, and the curing of women who have given birth."

As the historian Bridgette Sheridan asserts, these two title pages say a lot about the shifting nature of professional birthing care at the time, and the battle between men and women practitioners over who could best serve the wombs of France. Was it the traditional midwives, who had the practical experience and kept the propriety of the birth room as a women-only space— but were legally barred from the latest medical training because they were women? Was it the surgeons, who became masters of the new forceps technology in their male-centric vocation, but who weren't considered to be actual doctors and didn't know how to handle births without surgical intervention? Or was it the physicians, who were beginning to form specialties related to women's medicine, despite the social stigma surrounding male doctors intimately examining women? The ramifications were more than just financial; they would also change the course of medical caregiving—defining who was considered part of the budding profession, and who would be swept aside as folk healers.

A lot had changed between the birth of the dauphin in 1601 and 1627. After the assassination of King Henry IV, while Louis XIII was a child, Marie de Médicis reigned as regent. When Louis XIII reached his teenage years, he banished his mother from the kingdom and had many of her Italian advisers killed. Meanwhile, Louis XIII became France's first absolute monarch and welcomed his mother Marie de Médicis back from exile. It was in these heady conditions that a now sixty-four-year-old Louise Bourgeois served as midwife for Princess Marie de Bourbon-Montpensier, Louis's sister-in-law. A few days later, the princess died.

Marie de Médicis ordered an autopsy of Princess Marie, and the reporting physicians and surgeons (but no midwives) said that her death was caused by a small portion of the placenta that remained in the princess's womb. In those days, autopsy reports were rarely published, but in this case the physicians circulated their one-page report at court and disseminated it publicly around Paris as well. Bourgeois felt the blame for the princess's death was being laid at her feet, so she took the unprecedented action of issuing her own retort. She said the princess showed gangrene from a previous infection that her physicians should have caught (a diagnosis that modern historians agree was likely acute peritonitis) and that those physicians and surgeons in attendance at the birth—including the court surgeon Charles Guillemeau—saw that the placenta was delivered intact.

"Based on your report," Bourgeois wrote, "you reveal that you understand nothing at all about the placenta and the womb of a woman, either before or after her delivery; no more than your Master Galen [the then-unimpeachable Roman master of medicine for more than a thousand years], who had never been married, and having rarely assisted women in their delivery . . . it appeared that he had never known the womb of a pregnant woman, nor her placenta." Better for the physicians to look even further back to the ancient Greek physician Hippocrates, whom Bourgeois deemed smart enough to defer to the expertise of the *sages-femmes* "to know the secrets of the maladies of women."

For a woman—let alone a midwife—to make this move was a huge affront to the court physicians and surgeons, who immediately issued their *Remonstrance*. Though it was anonymous, historians attribute the writing to Charles Guillemeau, who went in for the kill: "You should rather have spent the rest of your life without speaking, than to claim as you do . . . that this great Princess was not as well taken care of as she should have been . . . Consider these things . . . and contain yourself within the limits of your duty—no longer involve yourself in correcting Physicians."

The surgeons and physicians ruined the reputation of France's most famous midwife and she retreated from court, where she quietly began working on her final book, *Recueil des secrets* (Collection of Secrets). Rather than focusing on birthing babies, it was more of a general collection of folk remedies she had found effective during the course of her long career.* Bourgeois published this final book in 1635 and died the following year.

Even in this time before the birth of clinical medicine, physicians in France had motivations both economic and social for separating themselves from healers without university degrees. Midwives were particularly easy targets. Few had the medical training and royal patrons of Louise Bourgeois.

---

* I was particularly intrigued by her "preservatif infaillible pour la rage," which I first read as an "infallible prophylactic against rage," thinking that would have been useful to her in her interactions at court, until I looked it up and found in this case "rage" translated as "rabies." The cure involves mint and absinthe and a number of other herby concoctions harvested just before the full moon in the month of June, which does sound a bit like a calming tea.

Instead of being referred to as *sages-femmes*—as the mid-wives called themselves—they were often dubbed *vielles* (old women), a coded reference to the elderly former prostitutes and madams in the provinces who used their experience with female anatomy to assist in delivering babies. Some physicians, such as André du Breil of the University of Paris, even went so far as to write that most midwives were witches.

Meanwhile, the strengthening of artisan guilds and government bureaucracy in early modern France was edging women out of the economy. When the French Revolution abolished the guilds and established clinical medicine, the marginalization of female practitioners was complete, with doctors taking over as the birthers of babies and positioning themselves socially as gentlemen. By the time Bourgeois's *Recueil des secrets* entered John Stockton Hough's book collection, his position as a Western male doctor practicing in obstetrics was the rule, and women midwives like Bourgeois were the exception.

The effects of this shift trickle down to this day. Women medical practitioners are perceived as less competent and less confident than their male counterparts even when exhibiting the same nonverbal behaviors. When the gender of the patient and the clinician are the same, greater satisfaction is reported on both sides, but when they are mixed, problems arise, particularly when a man is the patient and a woman the doctor. The power dynamic can exacerbate latent sexist attitudes in male patients, who come to view their female clinicians as incompetent and less trustworthy, making them less likely to follow their doctors' medical advice. Here the male gaze compounds the clinical gaze; gender bias both discounts the abilities of women doctors and affects patient compliance with those doctors' orders. Women doctors experience sexist attitudes not only from their patients but from their colleagues as well. Of the nearly six thousand women doctors surveyed in 2017, a whopping 77.9 percent reported gender discrimination in the workplace, with a lot of their unfair treatment stemming from reactions to their *own* pregnancies. I can't help but wonder what Louise Bourgeois would make of all of this.

What was it about Bourgeois's final book—in which the chastised midwife retreated from her supremacy at court to compile general herbal cures—that made John Stockton Hough feel it was prime for binding in human skin? Why did he feel entitled to use a female patient's body in this way? Did it matter that the book he bound in Lynch's skin was not the groundbreaking work that brought Bourgeois to fame, but the one she wrote in seclusion after her career-ending disgrace?

Though it is very tempting to speculate on Hough's motivations, I wanted to avoid doing so, lest I fall into thinking similar to the Princeton librarian Paul Needham's reaction to the Harvard human skin book. This thought brought me back to the time I paid Needham a visit.

Scheide Library, a room tucked inside Princeton University's Firestone Library, felt more akin to how I imagined Dr. Hough's home library than a typical academic rare book library. The tasteful Persian rugs and the stained-glass windows were once in the book collector William Scheide's home before he donated the accoutrements along with his $300 million book collection, the largest book gift in Princeton's history. The glass bookcases secure an astonishing collection, including an original printing of the Declaration of Independence and Mozart,

Bach, and Beethoven music manuscripts handwritten by the composers.

Needham had agreed to meet with me, and we settled into two leather club chairs. I asked him when he had first heard of anthropodermic books, and he was off like a shot.

"I don't like the term 'anthropodermic' because I think it's sanitizing," Needham began. "They're 'books bound in human skin' and anything else is trying to euphemize and therefore deflect from the central fact." Needham's familiarity with the practice of binding books in human skin came from the creations of Dr. Bouland, the doctor who bound Harvard's human skin copy of *Des destinées de l'ame*, which Needham had described as a postmortem rape.

There were many examples of books bound in human skin that didn't involve women, I pointed out, and alluded to my discomfort with ascribing sexual intent to the doctor who created the book without having concrete proof—like a diary entry or a letter—to corroborate that motive.

"Of course he chose a woman," Needham argued. In his opinion, the fact that Bouland specifically called out the gender of the people who were made into leather for his books was enough to infer a motive: "I do consider that an attack on a dead female body." Our main area of disagreement was around intent: Did Hough intend to denigrate women with his creation, or was the dehumanizing act a by-product of his blithe disregard for the woman as a person? We eventually agreed that the impact was ultimately the same, regardless of his now unknowable intentions.

Needham earned his Ph.D. in medieval history at Harvard and spent many hours studying in the Houghton Library, where the first scientifically proven human skin book is kept.

He was offended by his alma mater's disinterest in giving him a platform to debate the ethical situation surrounding the human skin book on their blog. It shut down the conversation he was trying to foment. "I am pretty permanently unhappy with the Houghton Library," he said.

Needham viewed the removal and burial or cremation of human leather binding as not even rising to the level of destruction of a rare book. Because books before the mass-market publication era had always been subject to rebinding, he reasoned, there was nothing sacred about them in particular. I argued that the singularity of the material of the book made it important to preserve, as evidence of this abhorrent practice. We can't go back in time and stop anthropodermic books from being created, but since they exist, they have important lessons to teach us—if we're willing to reckon with their dark past and all that it tells us about the culture in which they were created. We are finding new ways of reckoning with this truth all the time. My research could never have existed if the physical evidence was destroyed before peptide mass fingerprinting testing was discovered. Who knows what else we might find out about these books if they continue to be cared for by librarians like us?

I brought up the case that Nicholson Baker cited in his book *Double Fold: Libraries and the Assault on Paper*. Baker was mortified that newspapers in library collections were routinely being poorly microfiched or digitized and the originals discarded. Besides the obvious problem of not being able to rescan the discarded originals with better technologies when they were invented, Baker found evidence of some unusual cases where the paper itself was historically important. In the mid-nineteenth century, European rag paper suppliers couldn't keep up with the demand from the ever-expanding American newspaper industry, and as the price of paper rose, entrepreneurs like the geologist Dr. Isaiah Deck began exploring paper alternatives—most curiously, tons of Egyptian mummy wrappings that were being plundered from ancient tombs. Such an outlandish idea could be dismissed as folly that never came to fruition if not for a note in the July 31, 1856, issue of the *Syracuse Daily Standard*: "Our Daily is now printed on paper made from rags imported directly from the land of the Pharaohs, on the banks of the Nile." Baker discovered that most of the places where he expected to find 1856 copies of the *Syracuse Daily Standard*—such as the Syracuse University Library and the Syracuse Public Library—had discarded their newsprint after they were stored on microfiche in 1972. He visited the storied mummy-printed newspapers at the beleaguered historical association that saved them from the landfill, and reported that "the pages of the *Daily Standard*'s mummy issue rattle when you turn them." Couldn't new or future scientific techniques—or future biocodicologists and historians interested in material culture, for that matter—uncover more about this esoteric practice and the culture in which it arose? Was it not our responsibility as librarians, I asked Needham, to preserve these objects for whatever avenues researchers might take?

"I agree that librarians have a responsibility toward preservation," Needham responded. But "libraries have violated this incessantly in terrible ways, so it's a little hard to stand firmly on the pedestal if you're only applying it in the case of one binding at Harvard, when you've destroyed or thrown away tens of thousands of items of historical interest," he countered. "Here it's not a question of destroying the entire object; it's not the binding in that sense, it's the covering on the binding."

As two collections librarians, we could agree on the challenges we face when deciding, from our limited vantage point, what libraries should keep and what they should toss. All libraries wrestle with financial and spatial concerns and how to weigh those very real concerns against the potential needs of future researchers.

I found Paul Needham to be an erudite and interesting man. As our conversation drew to a close, he saw my gaze drift to a table displaying a richly embossed book, complete with the nubbed brass bosses that are used to support books that are left open for long periods. He smiled and said, "Would you like to see the Gutenberg?"

In my travels I had seen maybe a dozen of these earliest printed Bibles, one of the most revered works in all of the rare book world—but always under glass. Some are printed on rag paper and others parchment; some are simple and some elaborately illuminated with illustrations. They are all special in their own way. I tried not to tear up as I caressed the five-hundred-year-old leather on the outside of the book and was delighted every time one of its color embellishments was revealed with the flip of a page. That moment was a gift from one passionate librarian to another, and it will be with me always.

A FEW MONTHS PRIOR I had been in London, seeking out the Bouland book that Needham found even more odious than *Des destinées de l'ame* at Harvard. Retracing the other book's history led me to its former owner, Annabel Geddes, who didn't want an anthropodermic book for her bookshelf or for a research institution. She'd wanted to make it the star of a different kind of show—the London Dungeon. Geddes was no longer alive and able to answer as to her motives, so I wanted to visit the dungeon to sense what she had in mind. I knew the perfect companion would be the medical historian Lindsey Fitzharris.

We were ushered into a photo area, where her head was nestled into the stocks and I was given an axe. "Why are you executing me in the stocks?" she asked, mugging for the camera. I'd come to expect this behavior from my smartass friend with a Ph.D. in history from Oxford.

Fitzharris and I were there to have some fun, but we also found ourselves applying our knowledge of the way women's bodies were exploited historically and continue to be exploited all over again for entertainment value. The Jack the Ripper storyline unfolded over many rooms, where actors warned us about the murders happening in Whitechapel. One lady of the night told us about all of the Ripper victims individually, while windows with photos of their actual corpses lit up during each story. We were both taken aback. "Imagine being murdered so horrifically," Fitzharris said, "and then decades later a picture of your dead body is amusing tourists." It was disturbing that we were given no warning—nothing really separated the theatrical experience we were having from the images of the actual mutilated corpses of murdered women. No one else on the tour seemed to bat an eye. Indeed, this would prove to be just another example of today's dark tourism surrounding the Whitechapel murders. Shortly after my visit, a new museum was unveiled in the London neighborhood previously terrorized by

Jack the Ripper. What was sold to locals as a museum celebrating the history of women in the East End turned out to be the Jack the Ripper Museum, celebrating the mythos surrounding a man who viciously gutted marginalized women. When the museum's new focus was revealed, locals cried foul. After our experience at the Dungeon, I completely understood why.

I moved away from the fetid dark of the London Dungeon and into a clean, bright rare book library to unpack the rest of the book's provenance. Annabel Geddes, the controversial woman who inspired this adventure, founded the London Dungeon in 1974, and she later went on to head the London Tourist Board. At a Bonhams auction, Geddes bought Dr. Bouland's other human skin book—this one that still hasn't been scientifically tested—which was formerly owned by the obstetrician Alistair Gunn. Geddes purchased *De integritatis & corruptionis virginum notis* (1623), a title roughly translating to "Notes Regarding the Integrity and Deflowering of Virgins," allegedly bound in a woman's skin, for possible display at the Dungeon. At least one of the Dungeon's skeletons was proven in 2011 to comprise real human bones, so I guess Geddes had an unusual commitment to the authenticity of her spooky encounters. In the museum's carnivalesque incarnation, I can't imagine the very real horror of such a book fighting for tourists' attention. An unassuming human skin book just doesn't have the showmanship of a human skeleton. Maybe Geddes realized that, too, and that is why she never displayed it during her decades of owning it, before selling *De integritatis & corruptionis virginum notis* to the massive medical historical library at the Wellcome Collection in London.

I was met in the lobby by Elma Brenner, the Wellcome's specialist in medieval and early modern medicine. She assured me that now that the book was at the Wellcome Library, it was treated with the utmost consideration. She was surprised to hear that some other librarians advocated for the destruction of such bindings.

"They're historical artifacts. They're evidence. The thing is, in most cases we don't know whose tissue it is, so there isn't anything we can do about that, except to treat them with respect as objects. I feel very respectful toward that book . . . I feel like there's a woman who was exploited in death, so it's better that the book is here where we can share as much information about it as possible and it's not voyeuristically on display." The Wellcome restricts access to those with legitimate research purposes. They guard it from the morbid curiosity of those thrill seekers eager to touch a true artifact of horror in the guise of a nondescript old book.

In 2002, the Wellcome team had the two alleged anthropodermic books in their collections visually inspected by the National Trust for Places of Historic Interest or Natural Beauty, a charity that protects the U.K.'s "special places" and cultural objects, which concluded from the follicle patterns on the leather that the Bouland book once owned by Geddes was bound in real human skin. I hope that, one day, the Wellcome will permit my team to confirm their results with peptide mass fingerprinting.

While the Bouland book raises concerns over the exploitation of women, the other book at the Wellcome is racially problematic. It was created as a pocketbook (not in the sense of a purse, but an actual pocket-size notebook) and was allegedly bound in the skin of Crispus Attucks, a Black man who was the first person to die in the American Revolution. The National Trust deemed it a fake.

In my experience, most of the books highlighting the race of a binding's skin do turn out to be frauds, though for a time I wasn't sure why this was the case. My attempt to find an answer sent me down a path that revealed the extent to which the medical profession had dehumanized people of color throughout American history. It also had me questioning more deeply my faith in the written historical record.

{ 6 }

THE LONG SHADOW OF
THE NIGHT DOCTORS

Based on the written historical record, most of what we know about Crispus Attucks regards his brutal murder by British soldiers. His was the first blood spilled in the 1770 skirmish that became known as the Boston Massacre, an incident often cited as the beginning of the American Revolution. Most sources agree that Attucks was born into enslavement in Framingham, Massachusetts, the son of an African, Prince Yonger, and a Native American, Nancy Attucks, who were both enslaved. He escaped when he was twenty-seven and worked as a whaler under the alias Michael Johnson. Reports vary as to his level of involvement in the confrontation with the British soldiers, whether it was a planned protest that he led or a confusing street brawl or somewhere in between. Even in this basic sketch of Attucks's life, there are conflicting historical accounts that call into question every single fact I've listed here so far.

Crispus Attucks and the four other men who died during

the massacre—along with a boy who died a few weeks earlier, also in a skirmish with British troops—share a grave in Boston's Granary Burying Ground, the same cemetery where Benjamin Franklin's parents and multiple signers of the Declaration of Independence are buried. I thought about the small footprint of colonial life as I made the short walk from Attucks's grave marker over to the 1888 monument on Boston Common honoring the five killed in the massacre. A twenty-five-foot-tall statue of a woman representing the Spirit of the Revolution, with broken chains to evoke her liberation, towered overhead. The triumph of this imagery dissipated for me when I lowered my gaze to the bronze plaque at eye level, where Attucks's lifeless body was depicted. Even in his memorialization, it's Attucks's corporeal form and the meaning of his death—not his life—that's on display.

We know far more about Henry Wellcome, the nineteenth-century pharmaceutical magnate who bought a pocketbook with the label "The cover of this book is made of Tanned Skin from the Negro whose Execution caused the War of Independence." We know that after founding his American pharmaceutical company in 1880, Wellcome earned an incalculable fortune through the sale of "compressed medicines" that delivered cures in safer, more standardized doses than pills created using mortar and pestle. He even coined the word *tabloid* to describe the pills. He used his fortunes to amass the largest private museum collection in the world, employing a small army of agents to aid him in acquiring as many objects as possible from disparate time periods and regions. Despite his profligate spending, he kept a fastidious eye on all of his artifact transactions and was vigilant regarding fakes (though he was happy to commission a replica if an original was not for sale, should it fill a perceived hole in his collection). Despite Wellcome's attention to the origins of each piece he acquired, the Crispus Attucks human skin book apparently did not register as a potential fraud.

Scientific testing of leather was not available in 1929 when Wellcome purchased the book for £3—roughly $170 today—which strikes me as a low sum for an eighteenth-century book claiming to be bound in the skin of a historically important figure, though I guess the singularity of such an object would make it hard to comparison shop. If his agents had suspicions about its authenticity, they would have used the same visual inspection of follicle patterns that antiquarian book dealers have always employed, a visual inspection similar to the one that the National Trust carried out in 2002. Yet the National Trust determined that the Attucks book was fake. As Christopher Calnan, an adviser on conservation of organic material, wrote in a letter to the Wellcome Trust regarding the Attucks book, "The hair follicle pattern consisted of a set of 3–4 primary holes surrounded by smaller secondaries. The grain pattern was not flat but had a pronounced raised grain in between the hair follicles. The bookbinding is not from human skin. The skin has characteristics of camel, horse or goatskin. A heavy wax (?) dressing which fills the grain makes identification difficult."*

My team hasn't tested the Wellcome's alleged anthropodermic books through peptide mass fingerprinting, but when I held the pocketbook in my hand, with its pitch-black pebbled cover and metal decorations with heart- and moon-shaped cutouts, I was inclined to agree with Calnan's assessment. The leather on the notebook reminded me a lot of the UC Berkeley French prayer book that was proven to be horse leather, but my

---

* The question mark in parentheses is original to Calnan's letter.

gut had been wrong in the past. There's truly only one way to find out, and that's testing it.

Perhaps contributing to my initial skeptical assessment is that this book simply *irks* me. I find preposterous the idea that someone would hold on to Crispus Attucks's skin—from the Colonial American period, whence no other human skin book claims arise—and make this six-page notebook out of it. I have a hard time conceiving of why someone would ascribe this distinction to a book, why a discerning collector like Henry Wellcome would buy it, and—if it's indeed a fake, as Calnan and I suspect—why someone would fake such a thing.

The idea that someone would try to trick collectors and museums about the true nature of an object fills me with a mix of fear, fascination, and disgust. Art forgers are often motivated by a desire for revenge over their lack of success in the art world; they want to get caught, to prove their talent and cleverness, and money is only a secondary incentive. That motivation applies specifically to forgery: the wholesale creation of a new artwork that is purported to have been made by someone else. Divorced from a strong connection to a single creator, human skin book frauds could deceive collectors via a number of simpler confidence tricks, including adding a fake note inside the book's flyleaf claiming a human origin for its binding, or concocting a "provenance trap" in which the ownership story of a book gets changed over time to incorporate an anthropodermic twist.

To my mind, the most despicable kind of provenance trap involves someone leaving fake information about the origins of a book in a historical archive for researchers to find one day. Given how often I've come across a piece of anthropodermic book history in the archives that no one has written about before, the idea that my find could have been placed there by someone poisoning the historical record just to corroborate their fake story turns my stomach. Regardless of how a false anthropodermic claim gets attached to a book, the motivation seems to me to be purely financial; anthropodermic books sell for many times the price of the same book in a normal leather binding. The most puzzling element I've run across is the frequency of false claims about race among these frauds.

I WENT TO the University of Notre Dame to see another book, this one with a dubious note claiming it was bound in the skin of a Moorish chieftain. When I entered the gate at Notre Dame, the first thing I saw was their cemetery, which made this death-positive researcher feel welcome. Maybe it was a flashback to catechism class, but as a lapsed Catholic I was a little nervous about coming to Notre Dame and poking around, asking about an alleged human skin book. I was afraid the staff at the Hesburgh Library would disapprove. I really shouldn't have worried. Perhaps it was their comfort with saints' relics, but their librarians seemed unperturbed by the idea they might have an anthropodermic book; one expressed shock that these books were even controversial.

I hadn't intended on coming to see a book with purported ties to Christopher Columbus *on* Columbus Day, but it seemed fitting that it worked out that way. I met up with the Hesburgh's special collections and conservation staff to talk about the *Opera Joannis Pici Mirandule*. Published in 1504, the *Opera* comprised the posthumous collected works of the Italian philosopher Giovanni Pico della Mirandola, whose *Oration on Human Dignity* would serve as a manifesto for Renaissance humanist ideals after his death in 1494. The yarn attached to the *Opera* was a doozy.

The special collections curator, George Rugg, told me that the book had belonged to a man named Sebastian Carroll Braganza de la Coralla. "So this fella at some point was living in the Quad Cities area," he began, "and he gave interviews with the press describing the provenance of this book, which is that there was some Spanish Cardinal Ximenes. He killed some Moor who was particularly antagonistic to [Spanish king and queen] Ferdinand and Isabella, and had the book bound in his skin, and that's the story. Then it passed into the hands of Columbus and then following Columbus's death it found its way to the New World."

"It's quite a tale," said Liz Dube, the conservator.

"Yeah, it sounds like just that to me—a tale," I replied. I was thoroughly enjoying the head-spinning story and the enthusiasm with which the librarians told it. I just didn't believe it could be true. I mean, a famous historical figure *and* a racial claim? This was beginning to sound familiar.

We had talked for almost an hour before I realized I hadn't even seen the book yet, so I asked Liz and George to put it on the cradle for me. Five hundred years had not been kind to this book. There was a huge crack most of the way down the spine. Bookworms (which is really the common name for hundreds of different beetles, moths, and other bugs who love to munch on the wood and glue of antiquarian books) had over time bored pencil-point-size holes through its paper, leather, and wooden boards. I imagined that the blind tooling lines and rosettes—made by applying a heated tool to dampened leather and leaving the indentations empty instead of filling them with gold—were once gorgeous, but now the decorations were barely visible against the yellowed and browned leather. "Some sort of rodent really found it tasty at some point in time," Dube said, pointing to bite marks around the front cover's edges.

To my abject horror, a square turn-of-the-twentieth-century newspaper article called "A Medieval Book" had been pasted right in the center of the front cover of the book. Reader, it got worse. I opened the cover to discover more newspaper articles pasted within the book, with the words "The Grim Literature of Human Skin" written in outlined letters at the top. My book-nerd rage almost made my head explode. Then I noticed that, in one of the articles, a sentence about the price a human skin book fetched at auction had been underlined. To my mind, this mark was the smoking gun in this fraud's motivation for attaching anthropodermic status to an already historically interesting and valuable book.

Turning another page, I noticed that some scrap vellum of medieval sheet music, with its telltale red lines and thick black text, was exposed by the crumbling binding. Bookbinders in the early printing age often reused scraps from other books, which are revealed to modern historians only when the book begins to fall apart. Next to the scrap was a handwritten note: "This old Tome is part of a library Collection of Books which once belonged to The Church + were acquired by means of the Robber Rights which War gives; they are now returned to The Church with the sole request that the donor and his deceased mother be remembered in the suffrages and orations of the Community. Gentle Reader in your Charity remember me. S.C. Braganza de la Coralla." I instantly felt that this man was the book-mangling, human-skin-book-story-inventing culprit.

"Do not get frightened at the name," Father Paul Foik wrote

in 1916 when he asked his friend to inquire with Coralla about purchasing the book for Notre Dame. "Be rather afraid of the man should you meet him." Months earlier, the seventy-four-year-old "adventurer" Sebastian Carroll Braganza de la Coralla had arranged to marry the teenage daughter of a Lithuanian janitor in Chicago. Soon after the girl's family moved in with Coralla, the parents died in a murder-suicide. Some newspaper reports claimed Coralla was the intended target of his father-in-law's bullets. Before this gruesome scene, Coralla was already known to local journalists as a crackpot who liked to publicly predict that ferocious earthquakes and volcanic eruptions would hit in unlikely places like Chicago. When one earthquake failed to materialize, the press jeered, "People went about their business in this city much as if Mr. Coralla were not in existence."

Coralla's story about the *Opera Joannis Pici Mirandule*, embellished with the connection to Christopher Columbus and the binding from the skin of a Moorish chieftain, was a naked attempt to add monetary value to the book. The putative evidence sloppily pasted into the book itself gave the best clues I've seen as to the motivations of an intentional faker of objects with anthropodermic provenance. Sometimes the lies work because they are so specific and there are elements of the object (in this case, its obvious age) that could lead one to believe all the elements of the story that come with it. Since provenance is often spotty or nonexistent with books, as compared to valuable fine art, there are far more opportunities for falsehoods to be attached to these books, and to stick.

"It could conceivably be the case, too, that there's a kernel of truth in these elaborate stories," George Rugg said, but he didn't believe the human skin claim either. "None of us tend to think that's the case here, because it doesn't conform to any traditions of books being bound in human skin and the story is so incredibly florid."

Liz Dube became interested in the origins of the book's leather about fifteen years ago, but found the follicle patterns hard to discern. When I visited, the staff at Hesburgh Library did not know whether the book was legitimately made of human skin, but shortly after, my team tested the book and revealed its cover to be pigskin. With one part of the myth exploded (and further research by Hesburgh librarians unraveling the rest), I still didn't understand why frauds like Coralla so often described the race of the person whose skin was claimed to have supplied the leather. Was the idea of binding in human skin so in line with the treatment of minorities that it just made more sense than the general truth of these books' medical origins? Did the fakers think a buyer who would purchase a human skin book would find leather made from a person of another race more appealing? To my knowledge, no anthropodermic book has ever mentioned Whiteness—perhaps because here, as so often elsewhere, Whiteness was assumed by default.

As I drove back past the leaf-littered cemetery and through the gates of Notre Dame, I mentally flipped through our database of alleged anthropodermic books, trying to recall if there were any other books where race was a factor.*

---

* There is one other alleged book at Temple University, Dale Carnegie's 1932 *Lincoln the Unknown*. Yes, that Dale Carnegie, of *How to Win Friends and Influence People* fame. The green binding has a small patch of brown leather where the title is on the spine. Inside a typed note reads, "The title leather is the human skin taken from the shin of a negro at a Baltimore Hospital and tanned by the Jewell Belting Company." Though I have visited the book, repeated attempts to contact Temple's librarians to test it have so far gone unanswered. When I visited in person, I was able to see the book, but none of the librarians or administrators were on hand to speak with me about it. If the alleged piece of human skin is only the pasted-down brown square, this book might be a very rare case in which removing a testing sample might prove impossible.

What about books by authors of color—why would someone bind those in human skin? We have confirmed two anthropodermic bindings on text written by one of the earliest
African American authors, Phillis Wheatley.

A WHO'S WHO of the Boston colonial gentry, including the
governor, lieutenant governor, and future signers of the Declaration of Independence, gathered at city hall in 1772 to interrogate the teenage Phillis Wheatley. Eighteen White men, mostly
Harvard-educated supporters of enslavement as an institution, came at the behest of her enslaver, John Wheatley, in
hopes that, prior to the publication of the first poetry book by
an African American woman, they could settle once and for all
whether the erudite poems written under her name could have
possibly come solely from the mind of a Black girl.

Eleven years earlier, the young girl was purchased to work
in the home of John Wheatley's wife, Susanna. She was stolen from her homeland of Senegambia in West Africa and
transported on a schooner called *Phillis*, after which she was
renamed. At Susanna's urging, her daughter taught Phillis
how to speak and read English; Phillis excelled immediately
at reading the most difficult passages of the Bible and then became well versed in the classics and the poetry of Alexander
Pope. At age fourteen she began writing her own poetry, which
she read aloud to the astonishment and delight of the Wheatley family and their friends. Despite the publication of her
poems in newspapers around the colonies, there was widespread disbelief that the girl could possibly have written the poetry herself. Of Phillis Wheatley, Thomas Jefferson said, "The
compositions published under her name are below the dignity

of criticism . . . Comparing them by their faculties of memory, reason, and imagination, it appears to me that in memory they are equal to whites, in reason much inferior, as I think one could scarcely be found capable of tracing and comprehending the investigations of Euclid; and that in imagination they are dull, tactless, and anomalous."

"Essentially," the historian Henry Louis Gates wrote of Phillis Wheatley and her trial, "she was auditioning for the humanity of the entire African people." By all surviving accounts, she responded with tremendous grace to the verbal exam administered by a roomful of rich White men. Despite the incredible odds stacked against her, the men left that day convinced that Phillis Wheatley was the sole author of her poems.

Even with the blessing of the White colonial elite, no American publisher would produce Wheatley's poetry, so one of the Wheatley sons brought Phillis to England, where she became the toast of the literati and her *Poems on Various Subjects, Religious and Moral* easily found a publisher. She also met Ben Franklin while there. She was gifted a fine Scottish printing of John Milton's *Paradise Lost* by Brook Watson, who would become Lord Mayor of London, and she almost had an audience with the king, until Susanna's illness ushered them home early. When Wheatley wrote a poem praising George Washington, he replied kindly, thanking her for such a lovely tribute written by "a person so favored by the Muses, and to whom nature has been so liberal and beneficent in her dispensations," and set up their future meeting. When Phillis Wheatley's book was published in 1773, the Wheatley family freed her.

Sadly, her fame did not translate into an easy living as one of only a handful of free Blacks in colonial Boston. She placed ads in Boston publications for years in an attempt to publish a second volume of poetry but was unsuccessful. She married John Peters, a free Black grocer who left her after the birth of their third child. None of Phillis's children survived infancy, and the third child died with her in a poorhouse. She was only thirty years old. After her death, her husband sold her copy of *Paradise Lost* to pay off his debts. That copy is now in Harvard's Houghton Library.

Anthropodermic books are rare enough, but Wheatley's *Poems* are the only known edition with multiple confirmed human skin copies.* The Wheatley human skin books are both from 1773—one is housed at the University of Cincinnati, the other at the Cincinnati Public Library. They were donated by the book collector Bertram Smith, proprietor of the Acres of Books stores in Cincinnati, Ohio, and Long Beach, California (the latter now sadly defunct, despite the science fiction author Ray Bradbury's heroic attempts to save his favorite bookstore).

There are no claims attached to the Wheatley anthropodermic books as to the race of the person associated with the books' bindings. This suggests that the human skin binding is probably not designed as a statement regarding the race of the author or her enslaved status. Still, I had to do my own digging; I wanted a better idea of why these anthropodermic copies came into being.

Inside one of the Wheatley books is a bookplate from the Charles F. Heartman Collection of Material Relating to Negro Culture. Charles Heartman was a German-born White man of letters whose Metuchen, New Jersey, home became a hub for wild literary parties in the 1920s. He was an editor, publisher,

---

* Brown University has two anthropodermic copies of *The Dance of Death*— nineteenth-century facsimiles of the medieval memento mori works with dancing skeletons—but they are from different time periods and printings.

and writer, but first and foremost, he was a book collector with a great interest in rare Americana. His dictatorial personality caused his daughter to characterize him as "a little fuehrer." Despite this nickname, Heartman was a liberal who wholly assimilated into American life and frequently spoke against his home country while establishing himself in the book business in World War I–era New York.

The Great Depression decimated Heartman's business, and he cast about for cheaper places to live and work. He ultimately fell in love with the South and determined he would encourage a more active book culture there. He bought a four-hundred-acre plot near Hattiesburg, Mississippi, and placed ads in the newspaper entreating other bookish people to come live and work on his utopian Book Farm. As great as that might sound, the Book Farm did not work out. Despite early interest from librarians and other intellectuals, no one ended up living with the Heartmans on the Book Farm. Maybe they got wind of Charles's tendency to wander the grounds in the nude.

Heartman found the book collections of Southern universities lacking, particularly in Southern history and the work of local authors. He began buying and selling widely in books pertaining to Southern culture and in African American works; he worried that the few written works by Black Americans would disappear. He believed that if he brought individual pieces of African Americana together, he could more easily sell them as collections to the institutions where he felt they belonged. He also created and sold reprints of the most fragile and important items, coedited broadsides about Phillis Wheatley, and created a bibliography of her works with the Harlem Renaissance writer Arthur Schomburg, who called Heartman "a man with a big heart, a noble mind, and of generous impulses" and admired him "for his democratic spirit." He created a collection of Wheatley's poems and letters including some on Japanese vellum to make them more collectible.

Heartman's archives at the University of Southern Mississippi Libraries include a 1934 invoice from the shop owned by the famous London bookbinder Joseph Zaehnsdorf, issued for binding three Wheatleys "using leather supplied" and returning a fourth untouched. The third bound copy was long believed to be held at Rutgers University, but they have no record of it reaching their collection. As the Rutgers special collections librarian Michael Joseph told our team chemist, Richard Hark, "For me, there was a certain frisson imagining we might have such a prodigy in our midst, and, although I do feel our collection is somehow diminished by its nonexistence, I'm certain some other anomaly will emerge to console us." The total cost for Zaehnsdorf's binding services was 4 pounds, 12 shillings, and 9 pence, a rough equivalent to just under $300 today. Combined with our testing results of the Wheatley books, this invoice proves human skin bookbinding was taking place as late as 1934.

I have evidence that Zaehnsdorf's company had bound other books in human skin, including what I consider to be the most beautiful anthropodermic bookbinding: Brown University's copy of an 1898 *Dance of Death* adorned with skulls, arrows, and crossed knuckle bones. Who knows how long this company or others used discreet phrases like "using leather supplied" to continue the practice after a time when collectors knew to be circumspect if they were going to create controversial objects.

I couldn't find records of a doctor who worked with Heartman to procure the human skin, and I couldn't determine from whom the skin was taken. Without that information it's impossible to paint a clear picture of the ethics involved in the creation of the Wheatley anthropodermic books. Heartman seemed to respect Wheatley's work and her important place in the canon of American literature and lamented her early demise. "The literary work of her life is small, far too small," he wrote. "I feel that much original talent lay hidden in the soul of this poet, and that the best work she was capable of, has been denied us." Given what I could glean from Heartman's writings and life's work, it appears likely that he had the Wheatley books bound in skin because he wanted to create collector's items using the rarest materials to bind one of the most important works in African American literature. Similar to his decision to print some of her poems on Japanese vellum, he made decisions to apply meaningless but expensive material embellishments to her work, and he saw both a cultural need for preservation and a financial opportunity for a new market. But that doesn't change the fact that he got that human skin binding from someone.

When I started researching the provenance of the Wheatley volumes, I braced myself, expecting to find some nefarious figure hiding in a dark archive that had overtly ill intentions toward Black people. That was my own prejudice at work—borne out of reactions to the time period, the region, and the power dynamics at play. But I remain wary of the historical truths that transpired but were never written down.

Our PMF tests thus far do not show human skin books that were expressly made from people of color. We also can't confirm the motives behind skin binding of works by authors of color; I don't want to assume this was an attempt to exert power, the way Needham described Bouland's power play regarding women. Still, I don't think I could ever say definitively that it never happened. The lives of the White collectors of these books—who were not famous by most definitions—are better documented in the written historical record than even the far more well-known Crispus Attucks and Phillis Wheatley. These White people, members of the collecting class, had the most access to publishing and created much of the written history of this country.

Kept from the dominant written culture, Black Americans used oral methods to pass important information. Through these channels, they told of lynchings where White mobs took home body parts as souvenirs—a trophy-taking practice that anthropologists see in cultures where strong class distinctions, sport hunting, and racism coexist. Some of these oral warnings were specific to the medical profession, like stories of the Night Doctors who would steal Black corpses (or, in some versions of the stories, even living children) for medical dissection. The particulars of the original incident would get distorted or exaggerated, as any oral report might. Nevertheless the message was clear: beware of White people—especially doctors—taking liberties with Black bodies, living or dead.

As the medical ethicist Harriet Washington brilliantly showed in her book *Medical Apartheid*, sometimes the best corroboration of the Black oral tradition came from White media channels that Whites assumed Blacks would never be able to access. Doctors openly placed ads in newspapers, seeking to buy sick and dying enslaved people for medical experimentation. The doctor and the enslaver had a mutually beneficial relationship in which the doctor made a lot of money from treating the enslaved. The enslaver was the actual patient in that his satisfaction with the medical services provided were what mattered, and the enslaved person was relegated to a "medical nonentity." This view of the Black patient set the stage for a perpetually fraught relationship between African Americans and the medical profession that has ripple effects to this day.

Further, the aforementioned lynching mementos often included photos, which didn't look much different from photos of medical school students standing alongside their flayed Black cadavers. "Fortunately, the facts recorded by researchers and scientists themselves, in medical journals, texts, speeches, and memoirs, buttress African American claims for several reasons," Washington wrote. "Until three or four decades ago, these researchers were speaking only to their like-minded peers— other whites, usually male and rarely of the lower classes. They could afford to be frank."

It would be impossible to list here the history of the endless indignities and abuses suffered by Black people at the hands of American physicians. The Tuskegee Syphilis Study—in which doctors told Black men they were being treated for syphilis when they were really given placebos for decades, resulting in lifelong illnesses, deaths, and the passing of infection to wives and children, even after the simple penicillin cure was discovered—is the most often cited, egregious example of this injustice, but it is far from the only one. The Black body was overrepresented on the anatomist's slab and in medical research until only quite recently. The weight of this history has been devastating to Black health in America, engendering an understandable reticence to see a doctor unless the situation has become dire, a phenomenon Washington calls "Black iatrophobia," or the fear of medical professionals and institutions.

Doctors' biases toward Black patients persist today. To take just one example, a 2016 study showed that an alarming number of White physicians reported believing falsehoods about Black bodies (for example, that Black people's skin is thicker than that of Whites). Those who endorsed false beliefs were more likely to make less accurate treatment recommendations for Black patients. The medical profession has a lot of work to do to gain trust within the Black community, and it needs to start with acknowledging both past and continuing problems and educating medical students and practicing clinicians alike.

The idea of a doctor creating a book bound in human skin might not seem as shocking to people who know this history. Conversely, the true origins of anthropodermic books tend to surprise those with markedly higher trust in the medical profession. As the University of San Diego health communication professor Jillian Tullis told me, she was relieved that I hadn't found any books made with the skin of a Black person, but it wouldn't surprise her at all if one were eventually discovered.

"There's a long history of White male doctors taking advantage of women and people of color in the name of science, and then taking credit for those contributions, erasing the history of the people who literally sacrificed their bodies," she said. "If you're not familiar with any of this history, you'll fall into the camp that's surprised by revelations about doctors and skin books. But if you take a moment and are really being honest with yourself about our history—a history that includes the ownership of other human beings, as seeing people of color as less than human—then the ownership of a human skin book is not really a very big leap."

In addition, underlying every recorded account are the many people whose stories scarcely or never make the written record. For every Dr. Joseph Leidy, there's an Albert Monroe

Wilson, a Black "janitor" working at the University of Pennsylvania around the same time, who was just one of the Black workers tasked with quietly aiding the cadaver trade in the anatomy schools. As we uncover the stories of the people involved in the practice of anthropodermic bibliopegy, we must remember that relying on what is available in the written record means there are some stories that will remain hidden in the dark. While sifting out the truth from the rumors and innuendo, we can't forget that sometimes rumors are the only dissemination method available to the powerless, and innuendo is the coded speech wherein those in power can allude to the unspeakable.

7

THE POSTMORTEM TRAVELS
OF WILLIAM CORDER

Ann Marten's premonitory dreams always featured her neighbor's Red Barn, which earned its moniker not because of the color of its boards but from the otherworldly glow it emitted at dusk. In the local East Anglian lore, this trick of the light set the spot apart as a place of ill omen— and also the perfect place for trysts. It had been almost a year since her stepdaughter Maria Marten left for the barn with her lover William Corder, the son of a wealthy farmer. Maria had one illegitimate child and had recently borne another by Corder, but the baby died very young and was buried in a nearby field. In 1820s England, unmarried coupling and childbearing were cause for arrest; Corder told the Martens that the constable was coming to arrest Maria for bearing children out of wedlock, and suggested she beat a hasty retreat to Ipswich with him to get legally married. "If I go to gaol," Maria reminded William Corder, "you shall go too."

To avoid being spotted on their journey to the courthouse,

Maria disguised herself in men's clothing, but for some reason kept on her earrings, the green handkerchief around her neck, and the small combs in her hair. She topped off the ensemble with a man's hat. Ann bade them farewell as they left from two separate doors and headed for the barn, where Corder said he had arranged for a carriage to meet them and take them to Ipswich.

Later, Maria's young brother George said that the day the couple supposedly departed, he saw Corder leave the barn alone, a pickaxe on his shoulder. Corder assured the Martens that the lad must be mistaken; it was surely a neighbor planting trees on the hill. Soon the neighbors took note of Maria's absence. Mrs. Stowe, who lived closest to the Red Barn and from whom Corder had borrowed a shovel, asked after Maria at harvest time when she saw Corder at home helping his mother. He assured her that Maria did not live very far away, despite numerous conflicting reports to the contrary.

Mrs. Stowe asked if Maria was likely to have any more children, now that they were supposedly married. "No, she is not," Corder replied, "Maria Marten will have no more children."

Taken aback, Mrs. Stowe replied, "Why not? She is still a very young woman."

"No," he said. "Believe me, she will have no more; she has had her number."

"Is she far from hence?" Mrs. Stowe asked again.

He answered, "No, she is not far from us: I can go to her whenever I like, and I know that when I am not with her, nobody else is."

When Maria had been gone a year, Ann still hadn't heard directly from her once. Corder kept in touch with Ann and her husband, Thomas Marten, either by letter or on visits back to his nearby family farm. Unusually for the daughter of a poor mole catcher, Maria knew how to read and write, so her family was distressed that she hadn't written a single letter home. At one point, Corder explained that she was afflicted by a growth on her hand that made it impossible for her to write; another time, he vowed to hold the post office responsible for losing a letter that he claimed Maria had sent to her father.

As time dragged on, Ann's horrible dreams intensified. Reluctantly, she brought her concerns to her husband: "I think, were I in your place, I would go and examine the Red Barn. I have very frequently dreamed about Maria, and twice before Christmas I dreamed that Maria was murdered and buried in the Red Barn."

Asked why she hadn't told him before, Ann said she was afraid that he would think she was being superstitious. Thomas Marten grabbed his mole spud—a sharp metal tool he used to kill the creatures in the ground—and made his way to the Red Barn. He began poking into its floors and soon noticed that the ground was softer where the corn harvest had recently been resting. He cleared away the earth to find the badly decomposed corpse of his daughter, green kerchief still tied stiflingly tight around her neck. Her combs and earrings were littered among the gore and exposed skeletal limbs.

He called the authorities, who did their best to assess the scene, despite not having the appropriate facilities or much experience with murder investigations in their tiny country village of Polstead. A local surgeon made notes of the state of Maria's body while she still lay in her shallow grave, then some men lifted her body onto a door to take her to the local pub for closer examination. In their attempt to move her, her rotting hand dropped onto the barn floor. They found signs of a gunshot wound to the face and other wounds consistent with stabbing, choking, or dragging. They concluded that someone would have to find William Corder right away.

In London, a police officer located him in the family home of his new wife, whom he had found after placing an ad in *The Times* lamenting the recent loss of the "chief of his family by the hand of Providence" and expressing his hope to find a suitable replacement. The officer asked Corder three times whether he knew someone named Maria Marten, and each time Corder assured him that he knew no such person. Soon enough, Corder was arrested and on his way home to stand trial for his crime.

Meanwhile, the sleepy towns of Polstead, where Corder's family lived, and Bury St. Edmunds, where the trial would be held, erupted with activity. Reporters flocked from all of the nearby towns and even from London to cover the inquest and trial. The brutal and salacious nature of the crime piqued villagers' curiosity. Near the Red Barn, a preacher drew a crowd of nearly five thousand onlookers as he decried the heinous acts of Corder, who already bore the new moniker "Corder the Murderer" in town gossip and folk song. Throngs of visitors were also entertained by a camera obscura and various impromptu plays depicting the crime in grisly detail. William Corder's mother had to threaten the playwrights over use of her son's name, as he had not yet stood trial—but still, "Corder" was on everyone's lips.

By the time the trial began on August 7, 1828, people from all walks of life had flooded Bury St. Edmunds in frenzied anticipation. Rain poured down on the umbrellas and bonnets of the gawkers; women were generally barred from entering the court, so they mashed their faces and dresses against the courtroom windows, reportedly breaking a few panes. Mischievous individuals passed the time by yelling, "He's coming! He's coming!," which would cause a fresh commotion until the spectators realized it was a false alarm. When the court officials arrived, they had considerable trouble getting through the unruly mob; some had their forensic wigs snatched and one even lost his gown. Finally Corder appeared, his youthful, freckled face floating above a beautiful corbeau surtout with a velvet collar, paired nattily with silk stockings and pumps.

The prosecution was damning on the first day of Corder's trial. The court proceedings had to pause periodically because of noisy riots outside, and beleaguered constables promised to imprison the instigators should they persist. When court adjourned for the day, enterprising onlookers (many of them women—propriety be damned) climbed ladders onto the roofs of nearby buildings to attempt to get a look at the prisoner. Women of all classes showed keen interest in the outcome of the trial; one upper-class woman told a reporter she was looking forward to witnessing the hanging of someone who so inhumanely butchered another woman. Their weight threatened to collapse the roof of the courthouse. As a result, the ban on women in the courtroom was lifted. Constables stayed on guard for more shenanigans from rowdy onlookers for the rest of the trial.

The next day, Corder mounted a weak defense. After denouncing his unfair treatment by the press, he claimed that a distraught Maria had shot herself in the aftermath of an argument. Prosecutors called his explanation ludicrous, given all of the other injuries on Marten's body. After deliberating for about twenty-five minutes, the jury returned a guilty verdict. Corder dropped his chin to his chest.

"William Corder," the lord chief baron began, adjusting his

wig, "It now becomes my most painful but necessary duty to announce to you the approaching end of your mortal career." Corder shook violently throughout the rest of the lord chief baron's speech, his jailers occasionally propping him up to the bar. "Nothing remains now for me to do, but to pass upon you the awful sentence of the law. That sentence is—that you be taken back to the prison from whence you came and that you be taken from thence on Monday next, to a place of execution and that you there be hanged by the neck until you are dead; and that your body shall afterwards be dissected and anatomised; and may the Lord God Almighty, of his infinite goodness, have mercy on your soul!" The lord chief baron left the courtroom immediately and stepped into a waiting carriage, while the jailers carried a sobbing Corder back to his cell.

The excitement of the trial gave way to the buzz of activity surrounding the execution. The habitual hanging tree would not do, as William Corder would have too far of a trip through the dense crowd from the jail to the tree, so workers burrowed a hole right through the side of the jail, putting a platform underneath the gallows that would drop out at the right moment.

Public executions were always charged events, but our usual image of mobs howling for the blood of the condemned is incomplete. Hanging offenses varied greatly, and riots sometimes erupted at the gallows as friends and family attempted to save their loved ones from the rope. This urgency was heightened by the knowledge that surgeons lay in wait to dissect the bodies of the worst criminals, a fate anathema to most people at the time. Eventually the association between dissection and murderers was so strong that it was very difficult to convince people to promise their bodies willingly to the cause of science.

Corder was so unpopular and his crime so heinous that no one was likely to risk their life to save his at the end. But with a crowd this size and a trial this tumultuous, the village officials had to take every conceivable precaution.

While the men building the gallows busted the bricks on the outside of the jail, Corder wrote his confession about shooting Maria Marten and burying her in the Red Barn. Come Monday, some ten thousand pairs of eyes were fixed on Corder as he stepped onto the scaffold. Corder scarcely had time to take in the beautiful rolling hills and evergreen forests surrounding the Bury St. Edmunds jail before his eyes were closed forever. After just a two-day trial, his short life was over. But his corpse's work—and the work of relic hunters—had only just begun.

As Corder's corpse was carried back into the prison, the crowd roiled; spectators clamored for pieces of the hanging rope, a typical souvenir of infamous executions. Contemporary journalists reported that one museum official had even traveled from Cambridge in hopes of buying it for his collection. For his part, the hangman confirmed slyly, "What I got, I got, and that's all I shall say except that that was a very good rope."

An hour after William Corder's death, the county surgeon, George Creed, was already slicing a long line down the center of his body, peeling back the skin to expose the chest muscles before laying the body out for the public to shuffle past and gawk at. This was a common practice at the time and part of the public humiliation of murderers implemented to deter future criminals. At least Corder's body still wore his silk stockings and trousers while thousands gawped at his flayed corpse. By early evening, the public's bloodthirst finally sated, the professionals swarmed upon Corder's corpse. Artists made death masks and phrenological plaster casts of his head. The enterprising hangman collected what remained of Corder's fine clothing and the naked cadaver was transferred to the county hospital in Suffolk.

The next day, medical students and anatomists fully dissected Corder, and since any part of a dead murderer was up for grabs to local doctors, it was likely that at this point they removed a sizeable piece of his skin to bind a book about his trial. Mention of this book is absent from even the most detailed contemporary accounts of Corder's story; that could be because Dr. Creed made it for his own personal collection, where it remained until he bequeathed it to a fellow doctor before it finally made its way into a public museum. Creed made an anatomical wet specimen out of Corder's heart, and began preparing his skeleton for eventual articulation and display in the hospital.

"Thus I shall be able to show visitors to our hospital," Creed wrote, "at distant periods, the skeleton, heart and cast of the outward features of the head and face of this horrid murderer."

Creed was so pleased with the head's pronounced bumps—they corresponded with phrenological ideas about the secretive, greedy, and destructive behavior that Corder exhibited in life—that he sent the cast to one of the leading lights in the phrenological world, Dr. Johann Spurzheim. "I had a great pleasure in finding, on my return from Paris, the cast of the murderer Corder," Spurzheim wrote warmly, "which you were so kind as to send for my collection, and for which I give you my best thanks." Aside from the alluring head bumps of great geniuses, phrenologists were most intrigued by what their then-popular pseudoscience could tell them about the inner workings of the most depraved murderers. In addition to Creed's findings, Spurzheim noted that Corder must have been a man of low self-esteem and inferior intellect, but he was much intrigued by Corder's oversize region of marvelousness, or inclination toward religiosity or superstition. "I should like to know some particulars of Corder's private life—concerning his large tune and imitation; whether and how they have been active for themselves, or in combination with amativeness—secretiveness and acquisitiveness. The great development of this marvelousness, too, excites my phrenological curiosity."

Just as Corder was being dismembered, so, too, was the Red Barn. Relic hunters stripped off souvenirs from the location of the crime and made them into snuff shoes (for storing tobacco) and other items. At a time when policing was just becoming a profession and shortly before the rise of the fiction detective story, newspapers and books breathlessly reported the worst crimes of the day. Cases like Corder's contributed to a collective desire to own physical mementos from famous murder scenes, now called murderabilia.

A complex mix of motivations can contribute to the psychological urge to collect murderabilia. With these objects, the murderer shifts from the consumer of other people's bodies to the one being consumed (both physically, as he is made into objects, and culturally, as he becomes the subject of pop cultural works such as plays or murder ballads). Owners of murderabilia feel a renewed sense of control, which may help to explain why so many women were avid spectators at Corder's trial, execution, and dissection. The "morbid gaze" that gawkers exhibited as they marched past Corder's opened body is the same that draws us to true crime today: the push-pull between repulsion and fascination with the corpse, mingled with a thirst for vengeance against violence, turns death into entertainment for the living.

To this day people gape at Corder's corpse—or at least alleged pieces of it—at the Moyse's Hall Museum in Bury St. Edmunds. Corder's skin book is just one of the English books from this time period that purport to be made from the hide of a murderer of women. At Bristol's M Shed museum, a supposed anthropodermic binding covers the 1821 trial transcript of John Horwood, who—after an escalating obsession and attacks, including throwing sulfuric acid—murdered Eliza Balsam with a rock while she was out on a walk. In Devon, the alleged hide of the rat catcher and wife poisoner George Cudmore covers *The Poetical Works of John Milton*. Where murderabilia is concerned, not even a plaster death mask can compete with the unique, horrific object that is the murderer's skin-bound book. When the object was once part of the murderer himself, his corpse is commodified, which scratches a psychological itch for revenge.

I went to see them all, as I made this macabre journey rife with stories of domestic violence, execution, and retribution throughout England. When I made it to Bury St. Edmunds, I wound my way down the same gentle slopes that met William Corder's final gaze on earth; now these hills are chockablock with sweet cottages and picturesque churches. Today the town square of Bury St. Edmunds presents a charming mix of old cobblestones and modern chain storefronts, anchored by an astonishing twelfth-century building.

This is the Moyse's Hall Museum, and its archway leads to a dark view of the local history. A giant stained glass window suspended on wires depicts a wolf hovering over the decapitated head of a king. A gibbet also hangs from the high, arched ceilings. Prior to their dissection, this man-shaped metal cage was the go-to additional punishment for those for whom death alone was deemed too kind: it allowed birds and other animals to devour the criminal's corpse, denying him what was considered a proper Christian burial (in which the whole body remains intact for physical resurrection come Judgment Day). An Act of Parliament in 1752 for "better preventing the horrid crime of murder" permitted dissection in place of the gibbet for the worst criminals. At a time when the death penalty was used liberally for crimes as minor as theft, the threat of the gibbet (and, later, dissection) was how the state singled out murder as exceptionally heinous.

I reluctantly passed by the exhibits of mummified cats and the "witch bottles" locals hid in the walls of their homes to ward off black magic. Ron Murrell, the heritage officer at the Moyse's Hall Museum, greeted me in front of the exhibit dedicated to the Red Barn murder, which occupied a sizeable area of the museum. I wanted to see how a small-town museum told the story of an infamous local murder that resulted in a probable human skin book.

Murrell showed me a painted ceramic figurine of the Red Barn, a lantern said to have been used to help find Maria Marten's body, Thomas Marten's mole spud, Corder's brace of pistols, Corder's death mask, and a shoe-shaped snuffbox made from a piece of the Red Barn. There were illustrations from newspapers at the time of the key players in the crime; because Maria had no portraits made when she was alive, Maria's sister acted as a model for Maria's newspaper portrait. On a glass shelf next to the disturbing piece of darkened leather made of Corder's scalp and ears lay the much more normal-looking book of his trial transcript, which was also believed to be made from his skin. The murder of Maria Marten was one of the biggest things ever to hit this lovely little town, and this macabre collection of relics attested to its importance to the folks of Bury St. Edmunds and Polstead. "People still come from parts all over the world," Murrell said.

The only piece of Corder missing from the exhibition was his skeleton. Murrell pointed to a life-size picture of the skeleton and a small picture of a nurse posing with it. After Corder's dissection, the skeleton was displayed in the Suffolk hospital until shortly after World War II. "They used to take the skeleton out to dances—the sort of gallows humor you get with nurses," Murrell explained.

That gallows humor goes hand-in-hand with the clinical gaze that often develops for people working in medicine. For centuries, the human skull had been used as a prop in portraiture, and by the 1840s—a few decades after the Corder dissection—portraits of physicians and medical students with the tools of their trade, including skulls and other bones, became popular among the gentleman doctoring class. As photography became ubiquitous, it sparked yet another way to represent those in the medical profession—the disturbing trend of the medical student dissection table photo. Some of these photos depicted grave-faced students next to flayed cadavers, but they often took on fanciful tones. One popular theme was "the Student's Dream," which depicted many corpses in various states of dissection surrounding a medical student asleep on the anatomy table. The clinical distancing on display in these irreverent interactions between students and cadavers—sword fighting with severed limbs; a nurse dancing with Corder's skeleton—was viewed within the profession as a rite of passage well into the twentieth century.

After spending over a century at the county hospital, William Corder's skeleton journeyed to the Hunterian in London, an anatomical museum run by the Royal College of Surgeons of England and named for the collection's original owner, the eighteenth-century anatomist John Hunter. At the Hunterian, Corder's skeleton was displayed as part of an exhibit of executed murderers' remains.

When the museum was renovated in the early 2000s, the officials there—including Simon Chaplin, now the director of culture and society at the Wellcome Trust—considered what to do with the skeleton. A woman named Linda Nessworthy came forward, claiming to be Corder's descendant; she asked for his skeleton so she could give it a proper burial. Museum officials did not want to give a whole skeleton (and former museum object) over to one person claiming descent, especially when others could emerge later. So the College of Surgeons agreed to arrange for Corder's cremation and hand over his ashes to Nessworthy as a representative of the family. After years of lobbying the museum, Nessworthy witnessed the cremation in 2004. "It was almost like we were giving him a service that would release him—that he was going home," she said.

Emboldened by her success, Nessworthy petitioned the St. Edmundsbury Borough Council, which runs the Moyse's Hall Museum, to have Corder's scalp and skin book returned to her as well. The Borough Council's committee voted unanimously to deny her request because she was related to Corder only through a previous marriage, and closer relatives in town preferred to keep the rest of Corder's remains right where they were.

How could two institutions housing parts of the same person come to such different conclusions?

Back in London, I had some research to do at the Wellcome Library. I could tell by the hustle and bustle of the staff that I was very lucky to snag a few minutes with Simon Chaplin. He had run major medical libraries and museums in the U.K. and was a key decision-maker when questions about treatment of human remains in those collections arose.

"Museums should make decisions based on their own criteria and their own circumstances," Chaplin said. "There's a qualitative difference between a book bound in human skin and a skeleton. The book has never been used for teaching anatomy—that's not what it's there for. It was created and kept for entirely different reasons. The skeleton had been acquired under the Anatomy Act for teaching and research. It had gone on display at a later stage, but ultimately the rationale for keeping the skeleton was about teaching and research, it wasn't about preserving a memento of William Corder." He said the priorities of an organization like the Royal College of Surgeons would be to preserve the skeleton if it were part of Hunter's original collection, but since Corder's skeleton doesn't offer much opportunity to learn more about the organization's history, there weren't strong reasons for keeping it.

I wondered if museums routinely came up with their own protocol for the deaccessioning and disposal of human remains as collection items, or if there were agreed-upon best practices in the field. Chaplin clarified: there are laws and ethical guidelines to be followed, yes, but within them lies a lot of latitude for individual museums to make the choices they feel most appropriate. "I'm very comfortable that the Royal College of Surgeons took one decision with William Corder's skeleton and the museum at Bury St. Edmunds might take an entirely different decision with regards to the book," he said. "You have to be sensitive to the contexts of the acquisition, the history, and the current circumstance of human remains in the place that they are, rather than saying there's a set of rules that we follow that says yes we can keep it, or no this should be buried, cremated, disposed of, deaccessioned, whatever you might want to do."

I found myself understanding the perspectives of pretty much everyone involved in the afterlife of William Corder: the small museum heritage officer so steeped in the lore surrounding the murder and its objects; the venerable medical museum bigwig tasked with making very difficult decisions involving human remains in his collections; the distant relative who became obsessed with getting Corder what she considered a proper burial; the Bury townsfolk who would rather keep their famous murderer in his historic context than move him to his victim's resting place.

And then there was my small stake in all of this, the hope that the Corder book would not be destroyed before it could be further studied. Technically we do not know for certain whether Corder's book, or any of the other allegedly murderer-derived books I saw in England, are actually made from human skin, because our team has not tested them yet. I frequently catch myself having to fight the tendency to refer to them in the same breath as the others that we have confirmed with scientific analysis, because the provenance of the alleged criminal anthropodermic books is so strong; they have the distinct line of ownership usually missing from older books. Because some of the books are trial transcripts, if they are real, we are better informed than usual about the lives of the people whose skin forms their binding. Just as fake Red Barn snuff shoes or pieces of Corder's hanging rope could have been floating around, so, too, could there have been some fake human skin books that purported to be made from a famous murderer. If those who seek to cremate these books succeed, scientific and historical facts about them will be irrevocably lost.

For now, just shy of two centuries after his execution, the remains of William Corder rest, albeit in a number of places. Corder's story is unusual for the sheer amount of moves and physical transformations his corpse has undergone over the years. But his initial fate—of being executed, anatomized, and (less common but not uniquely) bound into a book—was relatively common for a murderer in his day and age. That all changed the very year of Corder's execution, when two other Williams, Burke and Hare, committed murders that would alter the norms of procurement of anatomical specimens forever.

8

ECHOES OF TANNER'S CLOSE

William Burke stood alone on the scaffold in Edinburgh in January 1829, facing the roar of twenty-five thousand Scots howling for justice. "Burke him!" they screamed. "Burke him, give him no rope!" The spectators wanted Burke to face the same fate that he and his friend William Hare had inflicted on their sixteen victims: they wanted him smothered—and his body sold to anatomists for dissection.

William Hare and his wife took lodgers in their flat in the tenements near the leather tanneries, on an alley known as Tanner's Close. Sixteen of these lodgers were plied with drink, suffocated by one of the partners in crime, and then taken in a trunk to Surgeons' Square for sale. The method could not be identified as murder using contemporary forensic standards, and it delivered far fresher cadavers to the anatomists than grave robbing. Once Burke and Hare's crimes were uncovered, the public raged at the idea that these people—all poor, some elderly, many women, and one with intellectual disabilities—had not only been brutally murdered but had met the murderer's fate of dissection while the culprits turned a handsome profit for their crimes. "Burking Mania" infected the populace, sparking reports of attempted and threatened burkings.

Though Burke would hang that day and not suffer a burking, the crowd did get part of its wish. After a long struggle, he was cut down from the gallows. A crowd milled around the university buildings in the rain waiting for Burke's body to arrive, so the authorities bided their time until dark before transferring his corpse to Professor Alexander Monro at the University of Edinburgh for dissection.

Like William Corder's, Burke's body was publicly displayed and then death masks and other artistic renderings were made before his dissection. The blood was so copious during the dissection that, as one witness recalled, "the area of the classroom had the appearance of a butcher's slaughterhouse, from [blood] flowing down and being trodden upon." Someone on the scene—probably a student—penned this grisly note: "This is written in the blood of Wm. Burke, who was hanged at Edinburgh on 28th Jan. 1829 for the Murder of Mrs Campbell or Docherty. The blood was taken from his head on the 1st of Feb. 1829."

This note, Burke's skeleton, and his death mask are all owned by the University of Edinburgh. In the nearby Royal College of Surgeons of Edinburgh's Surgeons' Hall Museums is a worn dark-brown alleged anthropodermic book, stamped with BURKE'S SKIN POCKET BOOK. A pencil still sits inside it. The fact that I have not yet gotten to see in person this most famous of all the alleged human skin books eats me up inside. When I was skipping around the U.K. in search of skin books, the Surgeons' Hall Museums were closed for a £4 million renovation. While I was heartened to see that kind of dedication to the history of surgery, I will admit that I stomped my foot like a child when I found out that my European research trip was scheduled just a few months too early for their reopening.

In Burke and Hare's Edinburgh, it was a seller's market for corpses. Luckily for Professor Monro, he was the third in a line of Alexander Monros who had been anatomy professors at the University of Edinburgh, a position that secured them first crack at any bodies retrieved from the hangman's noose. Monro, who was commonly thought to rest on his family name, never updated his curriculum and charged high fees for the few dissection classes he could be bothered to offer at the university, even though hands-on dissection experience was required for students to be certified as surgeons. As Edinburgh became a hub of medical education, the legal supply couldn't come close to meeting the need for corpses. A younger generation of war-trained surgeons offering private classes found their services in high demand, and so did the body snatchers who illegally supplied surgeons with their course materials.

Even the most famous surgeons of Burke and Hare's time soiled their hands in this business. The legendary surgeon Robert Liston was an inveterate body snatcher during his student days. He read a newspaper article about a sailor's drowning and promptly piloted his boat to the small town in the Scottish countryside where the tragedy took place. After dark, accompanied by some fellow medical students, he reached the cemetery, where he saw the sailor's fiancée sobbing and dropping flowers on her lover's grave. After she left, the gang got to work. One of Liston's gravediggers even put one of the grieving woman's flowers in his lapel as they exhumed her sailor and made off with his corpse. As they pushed off from shore, they could see the woman running frantically back toward the disturbed gravesite, screaming and waving her arms at the scene she discovered. But by then the students were safely on their way.

For anatomists and medical students who could afford to pay, professional grave robbers—also known as resurrectionists—were a preferred source of cadavers. So when Burke and Hare found themselves in possession of a corpse, they also stumbled upon a long-established and willing market for it. One of their lodgers, a man named Donald, had died of natural causes while staying at Tanner's Close. Hare's wallet smarted from Donald's unpaid bills and the coffin he had been forced to purchase to bury him in; then the idea struck him that he could sell Donald to the anatomists to make up the difference. Hare and his accomplice refilled Donald's coffin with tanner's bark, interred the wood pieces, and took the body to Surgeons' Square.

Burke and Hare initially sought to sell their first cadaver to the same Professor Monro who would end up dissecting Burke, but, unable to find out where he lived, they sold to his rival Dr. Robert Knox instead. Dr. Knox offered them seven pounds ten shillings for Donald, an astronomical sum for the laborers. Younger, fresher corpses fetched more still—up to ten pounds, or two hundred shillings—which would equal one hundred days' pay for the hard physical labor to which Burke was accustomed. What had started as a bout of bad luck became a windfall for the duo, and soon they would find themselves in Surgeons' Square again.

Along came Joseph the Miller, who was sick and near death, so Burke and Hare decided to smother him with a pillow so his illness did not scare away the other lodgers. As they continued the killing streak that the press would later dub the West Port Murders, they refined their technique. Hare covered Abigail Simpson's mouth and nose with his hand while Burke laid his bulk across her body. It was this simple, quiet method, which left few signs and no murder weapon, that became known as burking. Burke and Hare never even dug up a grave. The pair made their way through their neighborhood's narrow pathways, lined with crumbling tenements, toting the night's kill in a large tea chest. Passing the sewage and blight, they eventually reached the airier, respectable environs of Surgeons' Square—and Dr. Knox's doorstep.

Knox was a Fellow of the Royal College of Surgeons of Edinburgh who ran lucrative and well-regarded anatomy and surgery classes out of Number 10 Surgeons' Square, serving more than four hundred students each winter. Smallpox-induced blindness had marred his left eye but did not affect his anatomical studies or his dissecting abilities. His theatrical style of teaching matched his style of dress, which was always at the height of fashion, with frills, lace, and diamond rings. Like the American Joseph Leidy, Knox felt more at home with dead patients than living ones, and he reveled in collecting and articulating pathological anatomical specimens. As Lisa Rosner wrote in her book *The Anatomy Murders*, "When a 'subject' was in the room, whether human or animal, mammalian, fish, or fowl, he had eyes for nothing else, and his many enterprises created a dangerously inexorable need for fresh cadavers."

"It seemed incredible to contemporaries that a respected medical man could connive at murder," Rosner wrote, "but it seemed equally incredible that he had no suspicions of the true nature of his purchases." In the most charitable view,

Knox's single-minded focus on acquiring fresh corpses prevented him from seeing the obvious signs of foul play on the bodies Burke and Hare brought him; for instance, they had clearly never been laid out for a funeral or buried. The fact that the anatomized victims were subsequently destroyed meant there was no evidence to use at trial against Burke and Hare. Ultimately Burke stood trial only for their final victim, Mary Docherty, and Hare was able to win immunity from prosecution altogether in exchange for testifying against Burke.

Knox thereby not only benefited from the crimes but destroyed evidence of them, and yet he was never brought up on charges. Knox was not even asked to testify at trial. His privilege as an elite physician allowed him to remain silent and to continue to practice anatomy as a free man, but he did not escape the ire of the public. Without legal recourse against the doctor, the people of Edinburgh created an effigy of Dr. Knox, parading it through the streets before hanging it in a tree across from his home. When that didn't satisfy the mob, they cut down the effigy, tried to light it on fire, and finally tore it to shreds.

Knox's colleagues did not enjoy the negative public attention that his association with Burke and Hare brought to their doors. Many of Knox's neighbors on Surgeons' Square believed he was implicated in the crimes. Sir Walter Scott objected to Knox's reading of a paper at the Royal Society of Edinburgh; the event was canceled. David Paterson, Knox's former doorman, who had routinely accepted the bodies brought to 10 Surgeons' Square, published an anonymous pamphlet, written by "The Echo of Surgeons Square," alleging that Burke and Hare had been encouraged to keep bringing Knox bodies for sale, and that Knox had ignored the visible signs of violence borne by some of those bodies.

A physician-led Committee of Investigation as to the Dealings of Dr. Knox with the West Port Murders, however, ultimately found that Knox was careless but not criminal in his negligence, and that he actually believed that the poor were habitually willing to sell their dead loved ones to the anatomists. Knox's students even presented him with a golden vase expressing their joy at his vindication and their sympathies for the hardship he had endured.

Despite the unwanted attention they brought to the darkest needs of the study of anatomy, the Burke and Hare murders helped change the law in the anatomists' favor. As the duo embarked on their murder spree in 1828, the Select Committee on Anatomy was preparing a report for the House of Commons. The last big change in British anatomy laws had passed in 1752, when an Act of Parliament gave judges the ability to rule that the body of a murderer be dissected by anatomists as a further punishment, in lieu of being locked in a gibbet like the one that hangs from the ceiling at the Moyse's Hall Museum. By dissecting murderers, doctors became agents of state punishment, and dissection a public performance of humiliation. The act was expressly described as a measure "better preventing the horrid crime of murder," dissection being seen as a fate worse than the gibbet, and with the added benefit, for anatomists, of greatly increasing the number of potential objects of study from the six cadavers per year previously allotted by law. In 1826, London's twelve anatomy schools reported that they had together dissected 592 bodies for the education of their 701 students.

The Select Committee for Anatomy was stacked with

followers of the Utilitarian philosopher Jeremy Bentham, a man who believed so ardently in the usefulness of the dead human body he insisted that, upon his own death, his be dissected by anatomists and then preserved. To this day (when he's not on tour) his seated corpse greets students at the University College of London. One French Benthamite passionately argued for the use of all of his body parts—including his tanned skin to cover an armchair for the Select Committee chairman Henry Warburton. Transcripts of the Select Committee's proceedings reveal that the Benthamites aimed to replace the limited pool of murderers' corpses with a more expansive one: the bodies of the poor in general.

The result was the 1829 "bill for preventing the unlawful disinterment of human bodies, and for regulating schools of anatomy." It stated that the bodies of those who died in poorhouses (also known as workhouses), or that went unclaimed by a suitable relative, would go to the anatomists. In their letter in support of the bill, the Royal College of Physicians of Edinburgh suggested as possible sources of cadavers "the bodies of persons found dead on the roads and streets, in rivers and canals, or the sea shore, in almshouses and elsewhere . . . as also the bodies of foreigners, strangers and others, dying at inns, lodging-houses and public institutions, in the absence of friends, and without visible means of defraying funeral expenses." Phrases referring to the "friendless" poor come up a lot in the contemporary discussions around the Anatomy Act. Imagine how friendless Britain's poor felt when their legislators sought to cut out the resurrectionist middleman and deliver their unburied corpses straight to the slab. Was this outcome even worse than the long-held fear of anatomists' digging up graves under the cover of night?

A few doctors called out the unfairness of the proposed act. The surgeon-anatomist G. J. Guthrie wrote to the home secretary in 1829 that it would be "a monstrous act of injustice to the poor of this country" if their bodies replaced those of murderers in his dissection room. He admitted he found the idea of being dissected repulsive, but continued: "If a medical man maintains the opinion that dissection is an unobjectionable process which people ought to submit the dead bodies of their friends to for the sake of science and the benefit of the living, I in my turn maintain, that they are bound to set the example." In a similar vein, the radical orator Henry Hunt suggested that if those living at the expense of the government should give up their corpses in exchange, then royalty should also be subjected to such a law:

> I would recommend, in the first place that the bodies of all our kings be dissected, instead of expending seven or eight hundred thousand pounds of the public money for their interment. Next, I would dissect all our hereditary legislators. After that, the bishops, with a host of those priests and vicars who feed themselves, and not their flocks . . . Were there a law passed to this effect, I would willingly consent that my body should be given "for the promotion of science."

That the elite found not only repugnant but absurd the argument that they should donate their *own* bodies for dissection shows the distance they cultivated between themselves and the poor.

Ultimately, some objected to the stealthy attempt to pass the bill; one letter in the medical journal *The Lancet* called it

"The Midnight Bill" for what the author saw as an attempt to usher it through Parliament without proper debate. Religious leaders acting on the behalf of the poor fomented enough distaste in the House of Lords to kill it.

Undeterred, the anatomy schools continued to pay for stolen corpses as usual. When resurrection men (never the doctors themselves) were arrested, the medical societies openly chastised the police for intervening in their cadaver supply. In their report to the Select Committee about the requirements and realities of surgical education, the Royal College of Surgeons wrote: "These interferences have usually only the effect of obstructing the progress of medical education, and of unnecessarily exasperating popular feeling and prejudice, without diminishing the evils or crimes which they are intended to prevent or punish." As modern policing began to take shape, the anatomists—imagining that their vocation put them above the law—resented being policed themselves. More often than not, though, their dissections went about unabated.

Despite his association with the Burke and Hare murders, Dr. Knox continued to conduct a brisk anatomy-lecturing business. The Edinburgh resurrectionists kept him supplied with corpses from as far away as Glasgow, Manchester, and Ireland. He even paid the wives of his most loyal resurrectionists to keep up the supply when their husbands were in jail. Then, in November 1831, another case of burking was reported in London, sparking renewed interest in reforming how anatomy schools procured their cadavers. Henry Warburton saw it as a fresh opportunity to try to pass his legislation.

This time around, Warburton rendered the tone of the legislation more palatable for the general public, shortening the name to "A Bill for Regulating Schools of Anatomy" and removing the mention of unlawful disinterment of human bodies. He replaced words such as "dissection" with "anatomical examination" and removed specific language that identified workhouses and hospitals as the sources of the bodies, though the implications were still clear. One major proposed change was that the bodies would no longer be anonymous; new rules required anatomists to report to their district inspector when and from whom they received a body, and the dead person's name, sex, age, and last residence, if known. If a doctor did not abide by the new Anatomy Act, he would face a fine (not to exceed fifty pounds) or up to three months in prison. The first version of the bill had included a punishment for grave robbing; this was absent in the second, signaling to doctors that if the act failed to produce enough corpses for their needs, they could feel free to revert to their old methods. "A Bill for Regulating Schools of Anatomy" was accepted by Parliament and became law in 1832.

Did this legislation render the creation of anthropodermic books illegal? Hardly. Assuming the book at the Royal College of Surgeons does, in fact, represent William Burke in the flesh, the circumstances around the legality of the book's binding are not addressed in the text of the law. In fact, the act deals only with *whole* dead bodies and doesn't mention body parts at all. It doesn't address the legality of making something out of the body parts exposed during dissection—be it a heart prepared as a wet specimen for anatomical study, or a piece of skin removed to bind a book.

The treatment of a body's parts versus the whole might seem a minor concern, but it matters a great deal in the eyes of the law. More perplexing still, legally a corpse was devoid of the rights given to a living human but was also not considered property. Stealing livestock could be punishable by hanging or deportation to a far-off penal colony, but stealing a human corpse was not a crime, because it was not a belonging. So while a lot of alleged human skin books derive from the era when murderers' corpses were anatomized, the 1832 Anatomy Act did nothing to expressly forbid the practice of creating anthropodermic books from cadavers.

The Anatomy Act was generally viewed by medical historians as a positive step toward supporting scientific medical education and diminishing the horrors of body snatching. When the librarian and researcher Ruth Richardson dug into the history of the Anatomy Act, she uncovered a more uncomfortable truth, which she details in her masterful book *Death, Dissection, and the Destitute*. As Richardson explained, "I had the ... difficult task of teasing out the rest of the story from the hero-worship most medical history represents." She continued: "The medical gospel according to the hagiographers horrified me—one long procession of Great Men—an ever-ascending line of evolution up to the glorious and smug enlightened present, with hardly even a nod towards patients and their experiences."

Richardson discovered that although the bill's main aim was to increase the supply of cadavers for dissection, it also took the seemingly contradictory step of making it illegal to dissect murderers' corpses. She saw this move as a deliberate attempt to distance the medical profession from the gallows, to diminish stigma around dissection and relieve anatomists of their status as the boogeymen of cautionary schoolyard rhymes. "There cannot have been much comfort to a pauper," wrote Richardson, "in the knowledge that he or she would be dissected on the slab *instead* of a murderer, rather than *alongside* one."

The act resulted in a greater class divide, with the doctors and their wealthy patients at the top, and the powerless poor at the bottom alongside the resurrectionists, who were maligned as "the lowest dregs of degradation" by the very doctors who filled their pockets.

The bill's writers also hoped to quell the anatomy riots that had occasionally erupted throughout the previous century. But another occurred just a few weeks after the passage of the Anatomy Act.

Cholera was spreading like wildfire across England in 1831, and those who died in the hospitals dedicated to cholera patients were prime candidates for the slab, as their families were well aware. But the government recommendations for cholera sufferers were that they either be sequestered in their own rooms at home with as few visitors as possible (often an impossibility in the cramped living situations of the urban poor) or try their luck at a cholera hospital like the one on Swan Street in Manchester.

In September 1832, rumors circulated that a three-year-old boy who died at the hospital had been maimed, and maybe even burked. Indeed, when his grandfather and a growing mob opened the boy's coffin, they found he had been decapitated and his head replaced with a brick. The mob paraded the open coffin through the streets and burned furniture along the way. Two thousand people rushed the gates of the hospital, and women roamed the wards in an attempt to rescue friends inside from a similar fate. Twelve men were arrested for rioting, and the board of health solicitor called for the arrest of the apothecary—the true culprit in the boy's beheading, according to the doctor who had tended to the boy at the hospital—but he fled, never to be seen again. The child's head was found among the apothecary's abandoned belongings, and it was sewn back onto his body before the boy was buried.

Incidents like this riot, and the overall reaction to the Anatomy Act, reinforced for the medical profession that the realities of their vocation were too harsh for common people's tastes, and that, therefore, secrecy was best. When some argued that Dr. Knox's refusal to speak publicly about the Burke and Hare murders was practically an admission of guilt, Knox replied that some eminent figures in his field had convinced him "that the disclosures of the most innocent proceedings even of the best-conducted dissecting-room must always shock the public and be injurious to science." It would be better for everyone, the doctors thought, if they kept the uncomfortable details of their educational needs to themselves; when infractions or ethical concerns arose, they would deal with them privately. As Richardson wrote in *Death, Dissection, and the Destitute*, "The indications are that throughout the nineteenth century, the surgical and administrative elites of Britain were prepared to turn a blind eye to (sometimes gross) breaches of decency and of the Act's regulations, so long as the public was kept in ignorance and the dissecting tables supplied."

The twentieth century saw a slow increase in body donations from people who—like Jeremy Bentham—had expressly made that choice. By the 1960s, between 70 and 100 percent of all bodies used for anatomical study in medical schools were donated consensually. Still, I was shocked when I first learned of how recently it became common practice to use donated cadavers rather than stolen ones. The idea of medical consent is so basic to us today that it's difficult to imagine a time before it existed. But indeed, all of the alleged examples of anthropodermic bibliopegy derive from the time prior to the midtwentieth century, an era when the concept of medical consent was codified into law (however unevenly applied). I was fascinated to discover that, around the same time Burke and Hare were terrorizing Tanner's Close, one American prisoner made a most unusual kind of body donation, and took the fate of his skin into his own hands.

{ 9 }

THE HIGHWAYMAN'S GIFT

Lying in wait, George Walton crouched by the roadside. Or was he Jonas Pierce now, or Burley Grove? It was hard for him to keep track. He had been discharged from prison just a few days prior to this December day in 1832, and had just a suit and twelve dollars to his name.

Walton used the money to buy two pistols with six-inch barrels, some ammunition, and the camblet coat with a high collar to keep him warm while he waited for hours alongside a Massachusetts turnpike. He had robbed some people as he made his way toward Boston, but hadn't secured a whole lot of money. He had high hopes about a man he saw in the market earlier, whose pocketbook was bursting with cash. Asking around town, he learned the man was from Chelsea. Walton was now loitering along the road to Chelsea, waiting for the man's wagon to pass so he could relieve him of that heavy pocketbook.

Walton was no stranger to the criminal life. He grew up

desperately poor in Lancaster, Massachusetts. When his mother died, his father left him with a grandparent, who also died shortly thereafter, so the child did chores for neighboring farmers to get by. When he was fourteen, he moved to Charlestown, Massachusetts, to find work. One day he helped a man carry a suspicious package and pocketed ten bucks for his service; he instantly found himself drawn to the easy money that crime could bring. Soon he learned how to make his way in the criminal world: which businesses were the best marks for robbery, how to spot the counterfeit bills that were rampant at the time, which stolen goods were the easiest to resell. He was first locked up at fifteen, for stealing cloth from a fishing boat, and was sentenced to six months in the local jail. "The idea of being in prison operated very painfully upon my feelings," he recalled, "I verily believe that if I had been discharged after the first week of confinement, I should have been honest and steady ever after. In a short time, however, jail scenes and the society of the depraved and vicious became familiar, and I lost, in a good degree, the tender feelings which influenced me on being first committed. There was so much mirth among those in confinement, that I soon became quite contented in my situation."

Whenever Walton got locked up, he resorted to every conceivable measure to escape. Over the years he dug tunnels, burned through wooden window bars, scaled walls under hails of gunfire, and sawed through leg shackles. "I never, in my life, was committed to jail when I had not tools secreted in my clothing or in some other perfectly safe place, which were sufficient to insure escape by sawing off bars, grates or in some other way," he wrote. After each attempt, Walton was recaptured, punished with solitary confinement, and forced to sleep on cold cell floors without a blanket, while the prison guards concocted new methods to thwart future escapes. But he outwitted them each time. Once, after getting caught digging through the floor again, Walton was moved to a cell in a disused upper floor of the prison, where he was chained to a ring-bolt in a corner of the room. Every day the guards checked that his shackles were secure. But Walton noticed right away that the metal ring was too big and he could easily slip his foot free, which he promptly did each day after the guards performed their inspection. He took advantage of these brief periods of freedom to exercise in his spacious cell, and on moonlit nights, he took great pleasure in sitting by the window of his private suite, gazing into the dark countryside.

Amazingly, given his propensity for escape, the twenty-one-year-old Walton was able to take advantage of a regime change in the prison system and garner a pardon in 1830. But his half-hearted attempts to find honest work at the Navy Yard, or ply one of the trades he learned in prison, kept falling flat. He also found himself running afoul of other criminals as he tried to become an upstanding citizen in the community. Once, he tried to stop a theft of a seamstress's purse and got stabbed in the head in a dark alley for his trouble. The knife penetrated three inches into Walton's head, and a witness had to pull it back out with his teeth since the handle broke off in the struggle. Walton somehow survived. Out of money and options, he rounded up old comrades from prison to help him plan a jewelry heist, or a scheme to run tobacco and messages back into the jail. "I did not go out of prison with feelings of a moral character, by any means," Walton explained. "I was determined to take any course that would most easily and readily fill my pockets."

So on that day in 1832, Walton was alone on the side of the

road, carefully eyeing the few wagons that passed. He hid his rented horse on a nearby lane and threw his cloak over the horse as camouflage. After more than two hours, the wagon carrying the man from Chelsea finally approached. Walton rushed up to grab the wagon horse's reins, brandished his pistol, and shouted, "Your money or your life!"

Normally his victims would fumble for their pocketbooks and give Walton whatever they carried, but this day, John Fenno, the man from Chelsea, gave Walton a surprise. Fenno sprang toward Walton and grabbed his shoulders. Walton thought he was just trying to escape, so he moved to the side to let him run, only to realize that Fenno was actually attacking him. Walton attempted to fire his pistol next to Fenno's ear to scare him off, but the pistol fired sooner than he'd hoped, and he shot Fenno in the chest. Walton fled back to his horse and rode away, looking back to check Fenno's state. When he saw the injured man rise to his feet, Walton was relieved that he hadn't killed him, and also rather impressed: "I thought, on his attacking me, that I had a different man to deal with from any I had previously met on the highway."

By 1837, Walton was behind bars again, this time at the Massachusetts state prison. The warden there, Charles Lincoln, was a creature of routine. Each morning he would leave his warden's quarters and patrol the prison yard; after breakfast he would patrol again. A devout man, he often visited the prison chapel around lunchtime to pray, then continued patrolling, including visits to the prison shops where inmates made shoes to sell. Eventually he'd retire to his room, where he meticulously recorded the day's events in his journal—which prisoners got punished with solitary confinement, which prisoners were transferred to other institutions, and which prisoners died.

During that summer, Walton got a minor mention in the warden's journal: "In Hosp. several times to see Walton who is very low and apparently near his end." This brief note merely scratches the surface of the time they must have spent together.

Walton wasn't your average prisoner—not only because of his swashbuckling escapes but also because, in spite of his slipperiness, he was liked by both his fellow prisoners and the prison staff. It is hard to imagine a state prison warden today taking the time to sit down with a single dying prisoner to record his life story from dictation, copying enough handwritten notes for thirty-two printed pages. But that is exactly what Lincoln did.

Walton caught the influenza that had been ravaging the prison populace, and his disease worsened into the "consumption" that would take his life on July 17, 1837. He died decades before doctors linked this wasting respiratory disease with the condition that afflicted Mary Lynch, now recognized as the disease called tuberculosis. In the close quarters of prison, infectious diseases like influenza and tuberculosis spread even more virulently than in civilian populations.

Lincoln must have spent hours at Walton's bedside, transcribing his tales of robbing civilians and fooling guards. Occasionally Lincoln interrupted the text of Walton's narrative with a bracketed aside, correcting Walton's recollections. For instance, Walton said that after he attempted to rob John Fenno, he lay low for a few days and that he "was not aware of being suspected." Lincoln broke in to disabuse the reader—if not Walton himself—of that belief: a friend of Fenno's heard the description of the perpetrator and "gave it as his opinion, that the villain was no other than George Walton and urged Mr. Fenno to take every necessary measure to ensure his arrest;

knowing that he was a bold, daring and reckless fellow and a very dangerous man to be at large in the community." Walton was in the middle of describing riding a stolen horse to meet an ex-con friend in 1835 when the warden interjected for the final time. "At this stage of the narrative," Lincoln wrote, "Walton being subjected to a severe cough, and feeling unable to continue any further dictation of the events of his life, requested it might be finished by those to whose authority he was subjected." Lincoln dutifully attempted to fill in the events that led to Walton's final arrest and detention in the Massachusetts state prison in November 1836, albeit with a lot less flair than Walton himself had employed.

Lincoln went to great lengths to bear witness to Walton's deathbed turn toward Christianity as well, a theme not alluded to at all in the rest of the account. Lincoln wrote that Walton's mind was poisoned early in life by "the infidel sentiments of some of the French writers" and that "he long entertained the dark notion of the eternal annihilation of the soul after death; and it was not until a few days prior to his decease, that brighter and more correct views flashed across his fading vision." The warden claimed that Walton told him that even from a merely selfish point of view, it would be better for a dying man to be a Christian than an infidel, that he wanted other prisoners to know that his mind was wracked with guilt over his life of crime, and that his fear of afterlife retribution had ushered in his newfound religious sentiments. We don't know whether Lincoln's account of Walton's change of heart is true, or just an attempt to convince readers that even this miscreant saw the merits of a virtuous life. But it was Walton's other deathbed wishes that ultimately made him immortal.

Despite growing up as a poor, orphaned farmhand, Walton

had learned to read and became quite a bookworm. When he wasn't trying to escape from prison, he read any book that he could get his hands on. He even read many books "of a religious and moral character," though those didn't seem to make much of an impression on him. I wonder if it was through his reading that he heard about the practice—transpiring mostly in the U.K. at this time—of binding the skin of executed criminals into books.

The prisoners who met this fate at the hands of the criminal justice system did not choose to be made into books—but Walton did. Although he didn't have his freedom, Walton took power over what happened to his body in death, just like he wrested control over his life by his many prison escapes. From my vantage point, he subverted a symbol of capital punishment by giving his consent to it. He got his incarcerators to bind two books in his skin, at their expense and his request. But I'll never know whether he saw it that way, or the real motivation behind his unusual bequest.

Shortly after Walton realized he was dying, he asked to see John Fenno, the man whose bravery had made such an impression on him during their stagecoach tussle five years prior. It is said that when the two met, it was Fenno who encouraged Walton to narrate his life story to the warden. We don't know what they discussed, but I'm left wondering whether Fenno influenced Walton's ultimate plan to have the attending physician remove enough skin from his back to provide the leather binding for his memoir.

The attending physician took the skin to a local tannery, where it was tanned to resemble gray deerskin, before sending it to the bookbinder Peter Low, who in turn bound the memoir and embellished its cover with a gold-tooled black leather rectangle that reads "Hic liber Waltonis cute compactus est" ("This book by Walton bound in [his] skin"). One of the copies of *Narrative of the Life of James Allen, Alias George Walton, Alias Jonas Pierce, Alias James H. York, Alias Burley Grove the Highwayman* was given to the doctor for his service; the other went to John Fenno as a token of Walton's esteem. The doctor's copy has never surfaced. Fenno's was kept in his family home for some time, where, according to family lore, it was used to spank naughty children and frighten them into good behavior.

Around 1864, Fenno's daughter, Mrs. H. M. Chapin, donated the book to the Boston Athenæum, where it remains today. The Athenæum, one of the oldest independent libraries in the United States, is also a subscription library where researchers can pay to access all of its materials on a regular basis. Those materials are impressive: more than one hundred thousand volumes of rare books, an equal number of art objects, a huge cache of original papers from the American Civil War, and a large portion of George Washington's original Mount Vernon library. Over the years, illustrious members of the Athenæum—from Nathaniel Hawthorne and Ralph Waldo Emerson to John and Ted Kennedy—have walked its halls and consulted its fine collections. Yet, often, people come here to see one book: the one bound in human skin. It's a distinction some of the staff have grown to resent.

The special collections reading room at the Boston Athenæum is not terribly large compared to the grandeur of the rest of the building's five floors, but it has very tall ceilings and a stately window with a lovely view. The walls are lined with giant bookcases of dark wood and glass, containing antiquarian books that actually look well used, far from the pristine gilt bindings of books designed to be seen and not read.

Walton's memoir was waiting for me there on a black velvet cradle—but not to be touched. Normally, researchers are allowed to hold rare books with their bare hands, but Athenæum conservators, concerned about the unusually frequent handling to which the book was subjected, implemented this rule. The library also digitized the entire contents of the book to provide more access to the work while preventing looky-loo visitors from touching it. The book was made with an "ooze" binding—an appropriately creepy-sounding bookbinding term for suede, or the underside of leather—that adds its own conservation issues. Suede is not as hardy as standard bookbinding leather, even when the animal of origin is not *Homo sapiens*.

In 2008, Stanley Cushing, then the curator of rare books at the Athenæum, appeared on the Travel Channel show *Mysteries of the Museum* to talk about the book. What he assumed was a one-off, minor strategy to help promote his collections ended up airing for years in reruns and then finding a new audience on Netflix. "You don't really want to be known for whatever freakish thing you own," Cushing told me. "I hope people have a wider net to throw about what intrigues them. People come in on Halloween and want to see it. That's not really who we are, please . . ." Cushing came to discover that the Walton story had more to do with who Cushing is than he had initially thought.

"He was a very handsome young man," Stanley Cushing said, looking at an 1820s oil painting of the warden Charles Lincoln that he had acquired for the Athenæum's collection. Lincoln had a gentle but angular face, not dissimilar from Cushing's own, though Lincoln never made it to Cushing's age. Lincoln was stabbed and killed by a prisoner named Abner Rogers, who was subsequently the first prisoner in the United States to be found not guilty by reason of insanity. Rogers was sent, by his request, to the State Lunatic Hospital at Worcester, where, within weeks, he threw himself out of a window.

A few years after Cushing acquired Lincoln's effects—including his journal and sword cane, broken during his murder but since repaired—for the Athenæum, he was doing his own genealogical research (a common hobby for librarians) and discovered that he and the warden Charles Lincoln are, in fact, distant cousins.

This is the kind of revelation that can come from doing research in person. Even when it had started to seem like the trip was a waste—being told I couldn't even open the Walton book; Cushing starting our conversation with a warning that he didn't have much more to say about the book than what he'd written in an article—an in-person chat with the guardians of these collections can unravel a completely unexpected yarn. Of course, it's crucial to consult supplemental digital materials before and after a visit, but there's a magic that occurs only when I put myself in a place and see what happens.

I've come to understand that my own experience as a researcher is part of a larger shift in the world of research libraries. As the book historian David Pearson put it in *Provenance Research in Book History*, institutions used to keep libraries to provide their users with access to texts. As master copies of many texts became available online, the importance of individual libraries holding on to those texts was called into question, and many have downsized their collections as a result. (Thus we librarians constantly have to field the annoying cocktail party question, "Aren't you worried you won't have a job now that everything's online?") However, around the same time, there has been a resurgence of research on the material culture and history of books. One hundred years ago, marks that showed former ownership were routinely cleaned out of old books; now, collectors perceive them to add value to a purchase. Books with markings made by famous people (called "association copies") are no longer the only such desirable copies; every doodle, bookplate, and underline in an individual copy could provide valuable information to scholars looking for clues to the ways our forebears read and what they valued. As of the past few decades, researchers increasingly travel to see institutions' individual copies of books with their unique markings and provenance. Pearson imagined a time in the not-too-distant future when "a twenty-first-century undergraduate textbook which has been covered with highlighter pen and marginal scribble may one day be valued more highly than the clean copy that some today might prefer." Of course, for me there is no book with more copy-specific allure than an anthropodermic book, especially one that an institution agrees to submit to testing.

Cushing didn't have any qualms about testing the Walton book to see if it was really human skin. "I see no reason not to," he said, "and if it fails, I wouldn't mind, because maybe not so many people would want to come in and see it from a freakish point of view." Unfortunately for Cushing, our peptide mass fingerprinting test concluded that the Walton book is indeed a real example of anthropodermic bibliopegy. Paradoxically, even though the Walton book's legend does not conform with any other anthropodermic origin story, its singularity made me suspect it was real. The book would not exist at all—no printer or publisher would have bothered to typeset and print just two copies of a memoir by an unknown highway robber—unless there had been some special circumstance. Walton seemed to want to ensure that his extraordinary life was matched with an extraordinary afterlife, and that both would be remembered.

If a prisoner is executed or dies of natural causes in America today, the exact fate of his corpse varies from state to state. Generally, if his family does not claim his body, he is buried at the state's expense in a prison cemetery. Often, no one attends these funerals, except for the fellow prisoners who are assigned to act as pallbearers or gravediggers for a person they may not have known. Finances sometimes force families to leave the responsibility for prisoners' remains to the state. As Franklin T. Wilson, an assistant professor of criminology at Indiana State University, told *The New York Times* in an article on Texas prisoner burials, "I think everyone assumes if you're in a prison cemetery, you're somehow the worst of the worst. But," he went on, "it's more of a reflection of your socioeconomic status. This is more of a case of if you're buried there, you're poor."

With Walton's unusual request, he made sure that he'd never be fully buried anywhere. He rests in the beautiful Italianate building of the Boston Athenæum, his skin forever encasing his life story. Reading Walton's digitized memoir, I couldn't help but be charmed by him. The experience of reading along, only to have his narration end so abruptly and be taken up by the officious Charles Lincoln, underlined the significance of the loss of his voice. George Walton was the only person we know of whose skin supplies an anthropodermic binding and who wished this end for himself, and the only one we get to hear about in his own beguiling words—not from those sentencing him to execution, as with William Corder's book, and not by the bibliophile doctors' brief identifying notes (like Leidy's soldier or Hough's and Bouland's women), but George Walton's life as told by George Walton. Maybe if he had lived long enough to dictate his story to its end, he would have shared why he chose this singular final disposition. But perhaps he did leave a clue in his *Narrative*: "The first law of nature is self preservation," he wrote, "and this principle would justify me in any measure necessary for the preservation of life."

{ 10 }

GHOSTS IN THE LIBRARY

On May 10, 1933, right-wing German students brandished torches as they tramped through public squares,
accompanied by marching bands. The marches were
organized by not the Nazi Party but the Deutsche Studentenschaft, an organization of German student groups, but the students and the Nazi Party had a shared goal: the suppression of
"un-German" literature. The Nazis had been dictating the
terms of acceptable art for years, even orchestrating stunts like
planting storm troopers, disguised in black tie, to boo Thomas
Mann at the 1930 ceremony celebrating his receipt of the Nobel
Prize.* The Studentenschaft march would culminate in a book-
burning in Berlin's Opernplatz.

The minister of propaganda, Joseph Goebbels, agreed to
give a speech for the forty thousand students assembled in

---

* It didn't matter, of course, that Mann was once right-wing and even coined the term
Third Reich; he'd had a change of heart and publicly denounced the Nazis, and for that
he had to be punished. He was eventually forced to flee the country.

Opernplatz, airing it on the radio and filming it for later screening in the nation's movie theaters. "No to decadence and moral corruption! Yes to decency and morality in family and state!" he bellowed by the light of the pyre. "I consign to the flames the writings of Heinrich Mann, Ernst Gläser, Erich Kästner."

On that day alone, these students burned more than twenty-five thousand books in their "fire oaths." Few of Berlin's libraries or other cultural institutions were safe. Earlier that week, one hundred of these students had ravaged the Institute of Sexual Studies (Institut für Sexualwissenschaft, or ISS), which conducted research that promoted the rights of women and gay and trans people; running amok in the ISS for hours, they destroyed as much as they could, breaking windows, pouring paint on the carpets, and stealing books and archival materials. By 11:00 p.m. on May 10, the students produced the sculpted head of Magnus Hirschfeld, the medical doctor who had founded the ISS, and paraded it through the streets. Hirschfeld's head soon joined the books on the pyre.

The banning and burning of books by Nazi groups persists as a chilling image and a warning of the horrors that would erupt from that regime; as the Nazi-banned author Heinrich Heine prophetically wrote in 1820, "Where they burn books, they will in the end also burn people." It also cemented the narrative of the Nazis as anti-intellectual brutes, all while a quieter cultural plunder was underway. The rioting students stole some of the books from the Institute for Sexual Studies, but not all of them: later, storm troopers impounded the more than ten thousand books that remained, as they did countless books at other libraries and institutions across the eventual war zone.

Hans Friedenthal must have heard about what befell his former workplace. Trained as a medical doctor, Friedenthal had led three departments relating to experimental biology, sexual biology, and anthropology at the ISS from 1919 to 1923, before leaving to found his own Center for Anthropology (Arbeitsstätte für Menschheitskunde) at the University of Berlin. His work focused on the heritability of physical and behavioral traits.

Understanding how genes worked in the evolutionary process, and, ultimately, how we could control them, was a major avenue for scientific research at the time, and while this led to important scientific advancements, it was also foundational to the eugenics and racial hygiene the Nazi regime would espouse. Studying variation was part of this line of inquiry, and Friedenthal was fascinated by the elements that made humans appear different from one another—for example, the softness of body hair in women as compared to men, or the reasons different races have different skin tones. He was particularly interested in how human and nonhuman animal hair and skin differs in its structure and appearance.

In 1926 he wrote that there was no scientific basis for viewing Jews as their own race, which obviously ran contrary to the philosophy of the rising Nazi Party. The work of Friedenthal's colleagues was dismissed as "Jewish science," even if the scientists themselves were not Jewish. Friedenthal did have Jewish ancestry; his family had converted from Judaism one hundred years prior during a wave of "Jewish emancipation," fueled by a desire to assimilate into society and avoid the social stigma caused by widespread anti-Semitism. His family's conversion was not enough to save him.

When the students ransacked the ISS in 1933 and the Nazis officially took power, Friedenthal was forced out of the University of Berlin. The year before, he sold to a London auction

house a very special book, a volume wrought with such intention that it remains difficult to imagine owning an object so
personalized only to sell it twenty years after having it made.

World War I had hit Friedenthal's family hard financially,
and perhaps his rare book made the journey that countless
others made during the era surrounding the two world wars,
from the library of a formerly prosperous European family to
an antiquarian bookseller or an auction house. A good deal
of these books ended up in American public institutions or
the private collection of an industrial robber baron. Some of
the greatest American libraries (like the Huntington Library,
Folger Shakespeare Library, and Harvard's Widener Library)
were greatly enriched by this influx.

We may never know why Hans Friedenthal sold his book
in 1932, but things went from bad to worse for him after that.
Forbidden to work in Germany, his adult children found ways
to emigrate, even if it meant months of internment in British
camps as "enemy aliens." His son Richard did go on to live a
long life in London as the respected biographer of some of Germany's most revered men, such as Martin Luther and Goethe.
It is unclear whether Friedenthal attempted to gain safe passage
for himself or if he thought he could weather the regime. Some
speculate that the seventy-two-year-old doctor was facing deportation by the Nazis when he killed himself in 1942, but as the
writer Ruth Franklin put it, in reference to other Jewish suicides
in the Holocaust era and beyond, "speculations about the motivations for suicide always have an air of ghoulish futility."

I went to visit Friedenthal's book at the Medical History
Center in Stanford University's Lane Medical Library. As
I flipped through its pages, I realized it was without a doubt
the strangest book I had ever seen. A dyed black leather cover

features a silver repoussé bookplate, meaning that the metal was hammered from the back to create a slightly raised three-dimensional design. The top of the square bookplate says "LADMIRAL," referring to the Dutch anatomical artist Jan l'Admiral, whose work is featured throughout the illustration-rich book. The center image is a profile of a Black man's face, partially overlapped with a skeleton's face peering in the same direction. Underneath are the words "Ex Libris Hans Friedenthal," the common ownership phrasing for bookplates to this day.

I've seen a lot of artist books, jeweled bindings, and other unusual materials, but I had never seen bespoke metalwork like this on the cover of a book, or a mark of ownership so prominent and in such an unusual format. Whoever commissioned the plate wanted all who saw it to know that this book was Hans Friedenthal's.

The inside cover has a metal border holding down an undulating mass of actual mole fur. Disintegrating silk endpapers of a purplish-brown hue have left deposits in the fur. The contents of the book are eighteenth-century pamphlets bound together, mostly works by the anatomist Bernhard Siegfried Albinus. One of them is entitled *De sede et caussa coloris Aethiopum et caeterorum hominum* (On the Seat and Cause of the Color of the Skin of Ethiopians and Other Peoples), which explains the book's cover portrait. One pamphlet features the iconic, playful fetal skeleton tableaus of Frederik Ruysch. But Jan l'Admiral's work is the main event. L'Admiral was one of the first people to print color in books by using copper plates to make three different impressions in red, blue, and yellow inks. The results are incomparably lush and velvety images that may or may not have caused me to utter aloud, "That flayed penis is just *beautiful*."

Almost overshadowed by this mind-boggling package is the writing, in pen on gray paper in the front of the book, that reads: "Dieses Buch wurde von mir in Menschenhaut gebunden, Berlin, 1 Juni, 1910, Paul Kersten," revealing that the German bookbinder Paul Kersten bound this volume in human skin in 1910, the latest date for the practice that I'd seen at the time.* A stamped message inside the cover takes things from bizarre to flat-out creepy. It translates as, "Think when you are terrified by humans . . . of your own human skin."

THE SHEER UNCANNINESS of Friedenthal's alleged anthropodermic book—and the fact that, the more I tried to learn about the book and those who made it, the murkier the story became—fascinated me in a way that no other book had.

Drew Bourn, the historical curator at the Stanford Medical History Center, was far less impressed. The way he saw it, the library's mission was to support research in the history of medicine, and very few researchers in that field were interested in the history of the book. Even for those with that combination of interests (cough, me), Bourn felt the library offered far more historically significant items, such as its large collection of Arabic medical texts ranging back to the thirteenth century. "This is one item out of many thousands of other rare books that we have, and they all have interesting characteristics in terms of their manufacture," Bourn said as he patiently showed me the Friedenthal book, "and if this is bound in human skin, then that's neither here nor there in terms of making it that

---

* It wasn't until later that I would find evidence that the Phillis Wheatley books were bound in 1934.

much more interesting than some of the other items in our collection."

But the bibliomaniacal heart wants what it wants. This book has become my white whale. I have spent too many late nights in German databases, cutting and pasting into Google Translate (and cursing my inability to read German), hoping to disentangle Hans Friedenthal's story, and wondering whether there just wasn't much to be found.

In 1910, Paul Kersten reported in a German book trade journal that he had bound six human skin volumes and a wallet during his career. "I was the first to be commissioned to bind books in human skin," he wrote, "which I obtained from a famous doctor and researcher in the field of the skin and hair of humans and mammals." Sure sounds like Friedenthal to me. Kersten went on: "These materials I tanned myself. I may therefore be considered competent and possessing exact knowledge in matters pertaining to how human leather looks, in its qualities and in its processing. I am therefore also qualified to correct what has been written falsely by others about human leather until now." He dismissed colleagues' assertions that human skin was indistinguishable from calf, and said it was far more like Morocco (goat) leather in thickness and most other attributes, though its deep follicles were more similar to pigskin.

Well respected for his artistry, Kersten worked leather in an expressionist manner that was later copied by acolytes. He was outspoken on all things, which sometimes put him at odds with the old guard in bookbinding, and caused him political trouble besides. He objected to the Nazis' impact on artistic license and quality in bookbinding; in 1931, he lamented that they had forced the German society of professional bookbinders Jakob-Krause-Bund to close, its economic problems worsened by the Nazi assertion that the field of bookbinding was run by Jews. Kersten was married to a Jewish woman and believed that Hitler's anti-Semitic discrimination appealed primarily to "politically immature" Germans. The Nazis launched a smear campaign, claiming Paul Kersten was also Jewish. His wife killed herself in 1943, and he died later that same year.

The weight of the dark stories bound up in this book became almost too much for me to bear. One night I stumbled upon a haunting photograph of Hans Friedenthal in the Landesarchiv Berlin. I stared at it for a very long time. I couldn't help but see suffering in his eyes. Each rumor I came across sent me down another fruitless research spiral. I simultaneously wanted to know everything about this book, to do justice to its history, and to be free from its grip.

Of course, I was dying to get this book tested by our Anthropodermic Book Project. Despite my increasingly desperate (and admittedly annoying) pleadings to the fine librarians who work at Stanford, they had no interest in testing the book, and that is well within their rights. There are many valid reasons an institution wouldn't want to perform testing like ours on their books. Some libraries and museums have strict policies preventing any testing that removes a piece of an object. Technically, even though the sampling size for peptide mass fingerprinting is so tiny that no one would ever notice the missing chunk, the method is destructive. Perhaps if some of the newest noninvasive methods work for our purposes, that could open previously closed research pathways for us. Some institutions don't want the attention that the testing and its results might bring. Our team shares results only if the institution agrees to it, though we do count every book from a public collection that we test among our total anonymized count. Still, some organizations would rather leave that genie in its bottle than risk potentially negative press.

In a more general sense, it is the library that owns the book, not the public, and most certainly not me. Drew Bourn was quick to respond to my questions, providing the most background material I had ever received from a librarian regarding an alleged anthropodermic book. But he was firm on the question of testing the book, and I fully respect that decision. Consent should be honored in all cases.

It was consent, after all—its historical evolution, its implications for medicine and in libraries, the ways it has been violated by people in power—that sparked my interest in the history of medicine in the first place.

I HAD JUST STARTED working at the University of Southern California's Norris Medical Library when a new faculty member called for the removal of Eduard Pernkopf's *Topographische Anatomie des Menschen* (*Topographical Anatomy of Man*, commonly referred to in English as Pernkopf's *Atlas*) from our collections, as he had done at the other institutions where he had taught, because of the book's associations with Nazi medicine. All librarians are familiar with the notion of a "challenge," or an attempt to get a book removed from a collection, which butts up against our aim of protecting the freedom to read. Hundreds of books are challenged each year, most of them written for children; the Harry Potter series remains one of the most frequently challenged, because of its alleged promotion of witchcraft. Book challenges rarely occur at the university level, and rarer still at an academic medical library, so I never expected to have to deal with such a situation in my own library.

The first edition of Pernkopf's *Atlas* was published in 1937 in Vienna. Its more than eight hundred anatomical drawings show the muscle fascia and other incredibly realistic details that were often missing from dissection illustrations. The anatomical drawings in the work were so useful to dissectors that it was printed well into the late twentieth century. Individual images from the book were republished in many other anatomical texts, often with some notable erasures: the SS lightning bolts and swastikas that some of the illustrators put next to their names. The marks did not appear in the copy in circulation at our library, which meant that the Nazi-medicine context in which these images were created had been removed from subsequent editions.

Scholars researching Pernkopf's *Atlas* in the 1980s and '90s concluded that there was no way of ever knowing whether the people whose bodies were depicted in the book were victims of the Nazi regime. Through the challenge process, it became clear to me that if books have to be removed from a medical library because the bodies depicted in them were obtained through unethical and nonconsensual means, there might not be an anatomical text left on the shelf. Beginning with the dawn of printing and modern anatomy in the fifteenth and sixteenth centuries and lasting all the way into the latter part of the twentieth century, this element of our medical history has always been with us. Doctors and medical students should know about and reckon with this aspect of their profession's history, and that is best accomplished by keeping the evidence and using it as a tool of instruction. For our library's part, we took our fight to keep the book in our collection to the Academic Senate. Ultimately we decided that the best way to address the issue was to put a plate in the front of the book and a note in the electronic catalog record, explaining the ethical issues surrounding the book and allowing readers to decide for themselves, knowing the potential origins of the cadavers, whether to make use of it.

We could never establish consent, but we restored the all-important context to the book, and also adapted it into a new teaching device, using the book as a focus for debate about ethics among medical students. Navigating the ethical implications surrounding the sourcing of bodies for anatomical instruction and publishing, and what my role could be in turning these uncomfortable issues into learning opportunities, made a huge impact on me early in my career. All of my work as a librarian, a writer, and a death-positive activist is rooted in the lessons the *Topographische Anatomie des Menschen* taught me. If that faculty member were successful in removing the book, these lessons would not have been possible.

At the time of this writing, no Pernkopf *Atlas* is anthropodermic, nor are any other books from that era. Yet when people hear that I study books bound in human skin, the first question I usually get is, "That's a Nazi thing, right?" My glib response used to be, "No, Nazis burned books. They didn't prize and collect them the way that those who created anthropodermic books did." As I researched further, though, I discovered that I was generalizing, much like the people who asked me that question. The incorrect part of my assumption was that because Nazis burned books, they didn't value them as sources of knowledge or as collectible objects (as they famously did fine art).

I was grossly mistaken. Nazis knew the value of controlling information and exercised their control through many means. Yes, they burned countless books. They also stole tens of millions of books. They repurposed collections of looted libraries as intellectual fodder for studying their enemies: Jews, Freemasons, Catholics, Poles, Bolsheviks, Rom, Jehovah's Witnesses, gay people. They planned to form research institutions across the Reichsland on the basis of these collections. The most sickening of all was the Institut zur Erforschung der Judenfrage, or the Institute for Research on the Jewish Question, which opened in Frankfurt in 1941. Though Nazi art collections got the most attention, book collecting also conferred status and was in keeping with the Nazis' totalitarian narcissism, positioning them as the owners and controllers of cherished objects, full of information from conquered cultures.

Heinrich Himmler's penchant for occult books was well known, and his library amassed works about theosophy, magical incantations, astrology, and other occult topics, often robbed from Freemasons' libraries. Like the swastikas removed from Pernkopf's *Atlas* illustrations, these books' contexts were erased—either by the books' removal from their original owners, or in some cases quite literally, by colluding librarians who erased or cut out ownership marks and bookplates. Other librarians heroically smuggled valuable texts out of the stolen libraries. Some librarians today, most notably Detlef Bockenkamm and Sebastian Finsterwalder at the Zentral- und Landesbibliothek, have attempted to find the original owners of the Nazi-plundered books that ended up in their library, building a searchable database where people can use identifying marks and bookplates to try to find the rightful owners. Their work is not as well supported as the efforts to repatriate Nazi stolen art, however, because the books are less valuable and showy.

I spent a few late nights searching this database myself and found one book owned by Richard Friedenthal, and another written by Hans Friedenthal and owned by an Oskar Hein who was murdered in the Holocaust. I sent the results of my rudimentary sleuthing to the team at Zentral- und Landesbibliothek in hopes that I could help get these books to their families of origin, but finding living descendants might still prove difficult, and the more time passes, the more difficult that task becomes. As Finsterwalder said, "These books are like ghosts in the library," relics of past lives disrupted, displaced, and whole lineages snuffed out.

I should have known better—just because I had never heard of Nazis plundering books didn't mean it never happened. It did happen, and on an unfathomable scale. The layering of atrocities during the Holocaust is so dense that such a holistic assault on the written culture could be relegated to a mere footnote. But as to whether the Nazis made books out of human skin, the short answer is that there is no proof of the practice as of this writing, but I can't be certain that an alleged human skin book won't eventually surface. If one does, each claim should be taken seriously and tested scientifically if possible. To understand why Nazis are the first association to leap to mind when considering human-skin-bound books, however, we must consider Germany's largest concentration camp: Buchenwald.

Buchenwald got its name from the surrounding forests, which secluded its horrors from public view. That forest would earn the nickname "the Singing Forest" because of the tortured moans that echoed from prisoners hanging from its trees. Many of the prisoners were artists and writers, including the eventual Nobel Laureate Elie Wiesel. A special ancient oak in the forest was named for another writer, whose legacy the Nazis were trying to subvert for their purposes: Johann

Wolfgang von Goethe, whose life Richard Friedenthal would later chronicle.

On April 16, 1945, a film was shot from a moving car rumbling down a road in this forest. Its skinny birch trees shaded dozens of German civilians—many of them smartly dressed women in jackets, skirts, and heels—walking roadside, some smiling, looking as though they were on a Sunday stroll. A passing Jeep emblazoned with the words MILITARY POLICE in English denoted that the pedestrians were under orders from the American military: they were being marched to Buchenwald to bear witness to the atrocities that had been committed in their midst. Some held handkerchiefs over their faces when confronted with a truck piled with emaciated corpses; others walked briskly by them with stern, avoidant eyes. A woman who fainted was carried out. Newly freed prisoners, still in their striped uniforms, stood behind barbed wire, watching them watch. Another scene showed a crowd, some heads in military helmets, with a few inches of a large lampshade just visible above them. Footage from another angle revealed that the lampshade was part of a display that included organs in jars, shrunken heads, and multiple pieces of preserved, tattooed skin. Some brittle, hardened pieces of skin, held down with rocks, rustled in the breeze. But it was the lampshade in this film that would come to occupy an unusual place in our collective memory of World War II atrocities.

This lamp became an outsize emblem of the brutality of the Nazi regime, as it was claimed to be made from human skin. A mythos grew about the camp commandant's wife, Ilse Koch—referred to as the "Bitch of Buchenwald" and "Lady of the Lampshades"—having articles made from human skin and selecting prisoners with interesting tattoos for that purpose.

These allegations came up at her trial in 1947 and her retrial in 1950 but were deemed both times to be unfounded. Nevertheless, the association persists to this day.

As Dr. Harry Stein, curator of the Buchenwald Memorial Site, explained it, credible witness testimony from multiple prisoner-physicians working in Buchenwald's pathological lab reported that the camp commandant, Karl-Otto Koch, and the SS doctors picked through some of the lab's tanned, tattooed skin to find suitable pieces for a human skin lampshade. Koch wanted it to complement a lamp base made of human foot bones, intended for his own birthday present in August 1941. The lamp made a big splash at his party, but was likely destroyed immediately after, as Koch was brought up on charges of corruption and disorderly exercise of power by the SS and was executed. The lamp could have been used against Koch as evidence of his abuses, so he probably had it dismantled or destroyed.

When Koch's house was searched again in 1943, there was no sign of the lamp. The lamp in the film footage from 1945 had neither tattoos nor a base of bone, and it disappeared before the items on display were tested for authenticity by the U.S. Army. It likely became clear that the lamp was made from animal skin and did not belong with the true human objects made in Buchenwald's pathology lab—like those shrunken heads, which were made solely to test the possibility of duplicating the methods described in an ethnographic account of a tribal practice. Perhaps the strange look of the lamp and the persisting tales about a human skin lampshade circulating at Buchenwald caused this other lamp to end up on the table in the confusion of the immediate liberation of the camp. Some of the human skin items entered into evidence at the Buchenwald trial—now stored in U.S. government collections in Washington, D.C.—were cut into trapezoids and had holes punched in them, signs of possible former use as part of a lampshade.

After Germany was split into West and East, the East's Museum for German History (Museum für Deutsche Geschichte) displayed a third lamp—a small, simple bedside lamp that was alleged by the former prisoner who donated it to the museum to be made from human skin—that stayed on permanent display through the 1980s. After the reunification of Germany, an inventory check including authenticity research deemed the former prisoner's claim about the lamp to be unfounded. Meanwhile the narrative of the Nazi human skin lampshade persisted for fifty years, with people remembering having seen photos or museum exhibits showing dubious items standing in as these artifacts.

Over time, other cultural stories mingled with these associations; there was the human skin lampshade and other macabre relics found in the home of the American serial killer Ed Gein in 1957, and Mark Jacobson's book *The Lampshade* (2010) described the discovery of an alleged Nazi-era human skin lampshade. If a reader picked up a hard copy of Jacobson's book today, it would still aver that the lampshade Jacobson discovered in post–Hurricane Katrina New Orleans was proven by DNA testing to be made from human skin. In a subsequent documentary about the book, a lab retested the object and found that it was cowskin; the first sample was contaminated with human DNA due to the way it was handled.

No wonder the public persists in connecting the idea of human skin books with Nazis. It's easier to believe that objects of human skin are made by monsters like Nazis and serial killers, not the well-respected doctors the likes of whom parents want their children to become someday. Sometimes these stories we tell ourselves are harmless, sometimes they are pernicious, but they are rarely the full truth.

"It's tricky because you have little bits of truth and then all this myth," said Patricia Heberer Rice, senior historian at the United States Holocaust Memorial Museum. As the people who were present during World War II reach the end of their lives, the historian's role of separating myths from the kernels of truth becomes even more important.

"Take human soap, for instance," Heberer Rice continued, citing another widespread, gruesome rumor. "It's possible that someone, somewhere, made that. But it comes from rumors of atrocities from the First World War. If the Nazis did it as policy, we would know, because they used human hair for felt and that was well documented. A lot of the myths obfuscate the truth." She continued: "The lampshade issue is different, because there seems to be real bits of truth there . . . With this, it's more about trying to pull all the facts from the myth, what's not so, what could be so, so we know what really happened. That's the most important thing."

THE ANTHROPODERMIC BOOK PROJECT'S work is shocking by nature, but nothing could have prepared the team for what happened in 2019. One of our team members was approached by a small Holocaust museum in the United States about testing another alleged Nazi-era human skin lamp that had been donated to the museum decades prior and hidden in a storage room ever since. No information survived about who had donated the lamp or the story associated with it. We all instantly agreed that we wanted to help the museum find out more about their lamp.

When I was forwarded an e-mail with pictures of the lamp, I recoiled with disgust. The base of the lamp was tarnished bronze-colored metal and badly damaged; the old-fashioned electrical cord was frayed, exposing the wires underneath. The lamp was short, squat, and in the shape of a C, with a disproportionately large conical lampshade on top. It reminded me of a Venus flytrap. The panels of the shade were the color of undyed leather and translucent enough for light to throw the shade's every tiny line and crack into relief. In addition to the lines were huge, hardened, veiny protuberances spiderwebbing unevenly across the shade. The six panels of the lampshade were whipstitched together with a thick cord I couldn't identify—some sort of early plastic, maybe? Either way, this lamp was absolutely repellent. It looked like set dressing for *The Silence of the Lambs*. The idea that it could be real human skin was horrifying.

I don't think the Anthropodermic Book Project team had ever rooted for one result over another before. This time, though, I suspect we all were hoping for a fake. At least, I know I was.

Because of team members' travel schedules, it would be a few weeks before we got results. I flinched a little at every e-mail notification until we got the answer: not only was this lampshade not human skin, it wasn't even made from an animal! It was cellulose—made from a plant. I was not the only one relieved by this finding. On the condition of anonymity, the person who asked for the lamp's test talked with me. He told me they had made plans about what they would do if it were real: they'd have a rabbi conduct a service and bury it in accordance with Jewish traditions, complete with a headstone.

"When we found out it wasn't real, we were ecstatic," he said. "We had the biggest smiles on our faces; we're talking three people in their sixties jumping around in a circle, we were so happy." I asked him whether they would consider displaying this lamp in the museum now and telling the story of getting it tested and all that they learned from it. He said they planned to keep it in storage, where it has always been.

I am inclined to agree with Heberer Rice's view that we can never wholly rule out the possibility that something happened somewhere during the war, but to date, we have never found a human skin book made by the Nazis. However, there was one more surprising allegation about a book from that time period.

We Were in Auschwitz—the earliest Holocaust memoir, published in 1946—featured writings by three Polish, non-Jewish survivors identified by their camp numbers, including one who was later identified as Tadeusz Borowski. The book's cover mimicked the prisoners' striped uniforms. Its publisher, Anatol Girs, also a survivor of the camps, made a number of unusual bindings for the book. His daughter Barbara showed these versions, including one bound with striped cloth presumably made from an actual Auschwitz prison uniform and "another in the black leather of an SS officer's uniform and ornamented with barbed wire," to the writer Ruth Franklin.

Franklin reported: "A final copy was bound in what looked like pale brown leather. Borowski's name and the title were stamped in gold, and the sides were handsomely decorated with curlicues. The material was marred, its shading uneven; on the back was a large mark that looked like a bruise. Her father, Barbara said, had told her the book was bound in human skin." How could the only known example of an alleged anthropodermic book from this era possibly be made not by Nazis but by survivors?

Further digging revealed that the book was not a copy of *We Were in Auschwitz* but of Borowski's long poem *Imiona Nurtu* (The Names of the Current), published by Anatol Girs at the end of 1945. Girs had encountered his fellow concentration camp inmate reciting poetry and promised Borowski that, should they both survive, Girs would publish his work. When the time came to make good on his promise, Girs had a hard time even finding sufficient type to set the poem in the bombed-out shell that was Munich, but in the end he was able to get three thousand copies printed by the F. Bruckmann printing company.* The copy Barbara Girs showed Franklin was dedicated from Borowski to Barbara's father. Anatol Girs often had copies of the books he designed bound in nice or artistic materials as keepsakes for himself, and this parchment-bound volume was one of them.

Barbara remembers that when she was a child, she saw her parents get into a disagreement over the book. She recalled her mother, who grew up on a farm, saying, "I don't think that's calfskin, because calves if you're raising them for skin, you don't beat them and leave bruises! I think it's human skin." Anatol Girs was horrified at the idea, but there was no way for them to either check the claim, or forget it once it had been uttered. When I talked to Barbara Girs about her book, I ventured that all the real human skin books that I knew about were very intentionally made; collectors did not end up with one by

---

* Strangely enough, the Bruckmanns and the "Salon Bruckmann" that they held in Munich were a key entrée for Hitler to the world of monied culture and industrialists that would ultimately assist his rise to power.

accident. I admitted that the bruise was disconcerting; I had never seen a marking so similar to a human bruise on a book's binding. We both agreed PMF testing was worthwhile. "That would put it to rest," she said.

Our PMF results concluded that the book was bound in rabbit skin, another first for the Anthropodermic Book Project.

JUST AS THE NAZIS coerced writers, professors, and librarians to do their bidding in ways systematic and banal, doctors, to an even larger extent, benefited from ideological alignment with the regime. The Nazi focus on biology attracted physicians to the National Socialist Physicians' League early and in droves. Before Hitler even took power, 6 percent of the entire profession in Germany had joined the group; by 1942, that number was above 50 percent. There were seven times more doctors than members of any other profession in the SS, and many physicians rose to become the heads of universities and other elite cultural institutions during the Nazi years. At the same time, doctors working in the camps, and outside researchers with access to inmates, had free rein to do what they pleased with a captive population of unprecedented size. Horrific, unethical medical experimentation on the human body's reactions to extreme circumstances resulted in many prisoners' excruciating deaths from altitude, cold, disease, chemical burns, and more.

The Doctors' Trial, beginning in December 1946, was the first of the postwar hearings regarding Nazi atrocities to take place at Nuremberg. In his opening remarks for the prosecution, Brigadier General Telford Taylor stressed that the twenty-three doctors on trial were not "perverts" but trained medical professionals who should be bound by ethics. He also wanted to disabuse the jury of the idea that it would have been possible to volunteer for medical experimentation in the context of the camps.

"In the tyranny that was Nazi Germany, no one could give such a consent to the medical agents of the State; everyone lived in fear and acted under duress," Taylor said. "I fervently hope that none of us here in the courtroom will have to suffer in silence while it is said on the part of these defendants that the wretched and helpless people whom they froze and drowned and burned and poisoned were volunteers."

Prosecutors relied on American physicians to set the standards for medical ethics by which the defendants should be judged. This decision became problematic, because the American doctors cited standards issued after the trial was already underway by organizations such as the American Medical Association. Other ideals they cited, like the Hippocratic Oath, were not wholly appropriate in the context of the trial, because the oath deals with the treatment of sick patients and not with nontherapeutic experimentation on healthy prisoners. Ironically, the strongest code for medical experimentation ethics had come from the Nazis themselves. The Reich Health Council's ethical guidelines stressed informed consent and concern over testing on vulnerable populations like children. The Nazi doctors either didn't consider the guidelines to have the force of law, or just chose to ignore them, and met no comeuppance from that refusal until their judgment at Nuremberg.

In their final ruling, the judges attempted to correct this dearth of established international guidelines for human experimentation by dictating a standard—and thereby putting the text into the canon of international law—that became known as the Nuremberg Code. Informed consent was its first and strongest principle: "The voluntary consent of the human subject is absolutely essential." In the Declarations of Helsinki that emerged in the following decades, the delineation between patient care and research not intended to treat people diminished, forming an overarching international ethical framework for medical research and experimentation. The interests of the doctor, or of the progress of science as a whole, could not trump the interests of the research subject. That's not to say this code hasn't been violated time and time again, but there was now a standard set, and its impact on the medical profession was global. The doctor's gaze upon the patient underwent another shift.

"The Nuremberg Code's response is to prohibit the objectification of the subject by requiring the subject's voluntary, competent, informed, and understanding consent," wrote the medical ethicists George Annas and Michael Grodin. "The post-Nuremberg challenge has been to realize and protect the individual humanity of the human subject of medical research while permitting medical experimentation and, thus, progress."

Like all the myths we tell ourselves, our notions about the primacy of consent have seeped into our current understanding of the world so seamlessly that the origin of the concept has become obscured. We act as though it has been this way all along, though, in fact, our laws have yet to reflect this relatively recent shift in our worldview.

MY CORPSE, MY CHOICE

My body is my journal, my tattoos are my story,'"
Charles Hamm recited as he beamed at me from
across the table at a Cleveland steakhouse. He was
quoting Johnny Depp, which, he told me during our 2015
meeting, he did daily.

Hamm, the founder of the National Association for the
Preservation of Skin Art (NAPSA)—the nonprofit organization behind SaveMyInk.com—was high on the attention his
newest venture was getting and the possibilities it had for tattoo
enthusiasts like himself. I was interested in talking to Hamm
about postmortem tattoo preservation, because I found it to
be the closest modern practice to historical anthropodermic
bibliopegy, and I wanted to know more about what it was like
to try to undertake such an enterprise in a world where consent
is king. Many of us assume that, as long as a person consents
to something in the form of a will or advance directive before

their death, anything can happen to a body after death, but the law doesn't necessarily reflect this viewpoint.

Hamm came to truly appreciate tattooing as an art form when he was in his fifties. He began covering his body with work from the best artists he could find. His tattoos are a source of pride and self-expression, if also a hindrance to his career in finance; in the conservative circles of midwestern financiers, he said that his tattoos cost him spots on some top executive boards. One time he was talking with a few friends about all the money and pain sunk into his skin art, and he quipped, "You know, I'm going to get cremated, and all this shit is gone." To which his friend replied: "I'll cut it the fuck off of you. Have your wife call me. I'll come and cut it off."

What started as a morbid joke gave Hamm an idea. He started working with some embalmers, tattoo artists, and a doctor, and, through a lot of trial and error, the team came up with a preservation technique they marketed through SaveMyInk.com and supported through the formation of NAPSA. But first they had to try the technique on real human skin, and they didn't want to use a donor corpse, because what if the process failed?

As it happened, Hamm had lost more than a hundred pounds over the years, so he took this most unusual of opportunities to experiment on himself. He found a plastic surgeon who was willing to comply with his strange request. The surgeon marked where he was going to remove some excess arm skin, then Hamm got those areas tattooed (one with a traditional "Mom" heart and banner, the other with the initials of one of the companies he founded). When the plastic surgeon removed the freshly tattooed extra flesh, Hamm immediately preserved the skin and sent it to his team for processing using their secret technique. The results were pristine, vibrant pieces of art that Hamm promptly mounted and framed.

The sterile beauty of these pieces mitigates any ick factor; they are a far cry from the dried cracker of a preserved tattoo that accidentally fell into my hand at Harvard's Countway Library. Nor do they resemble the wet specimen tattoos floating in jars at the Wellcome Collection in London, examples of a historical preservation method common for doctors who wanted to keep the rare tattoo they found on a cadaver. Doctors had collected those specimens without consent and from those who were on the margins of society—sailors, prisoners, asylum inmates—but Save My Ink's technique allowed for the tattooed people themselves to arrange to preserve their skin art for future generations.

A lot of people today may balk at the idea of binding a book in human skin, but many tattoo enthusiasts don't blink an eye at the idea of preserving skin art. An Amsterdam-based outfit called the Foundation of the Art and Science of Tattooing promises a tattoo preservation service similar to Hamm's approach, but in their case, the tattoo would become the property of their museum, available for long-term loan to the families of the deceased. The supermodel Kate Moss speculated publicly on the value of her original Lucien Freud back tattoos, as if they were something that could be sold. The Zürich tattoo parlor manager Tim Steiner went far enough to ink a deal: his back tattoo, by the Belgian artist Wim Delvoye, came with a contractual obligation that he sit on display in museums such as the Louvre and act as a living canvas for the work. Once Steiner dies, the skin on his back will be removed and displayed—just where will depend on the whims of the art's new owner. Delvoye titled the work *TIM*, and it (he?) was sold to the German art collector Rik Reinking in 2008 for 150,000 Euros. "My skin belongs to Rik Reinking now," said Steiner. "My back is the canvas, I am the temporary frame."

Objectifying as these transactions might appear, ethically they are a vast improvement from the preserved skin objects of yore. They are consensual and documented, although I have questions about whether some of these donation forms are truly legally binding. And again, consent does not always mean the act is legal, and assessing the legality of the preservation of human skin—whether as a tattoo or to be made into a book—is not as easy to determine as you might think; a lot depends on where you're physically located when you shuffle off this mortal coil.

Charles Hamm told me that NAPSA looked at all the state laws in the United States and his counsel felt comfortable they were operating within legal confines. "Can I tell you that there won't be a state that challenges us? No, I can't tell you that," Hamm said, "but we're prepared to fight that."

I wish this issue were battled out in court, if only to get some clear legal precedence in writing. Although there is no federal law in the United States that specifically forbids preserving a tattoo on human skin, there are a lot of state laws that could be invoked to prosecute a group like Charles Hamm's or any of the multitude of groups offering to make your cremated remains into jewelry, press them into a vinyl record, build an artificial coral reef out of them, or any of the other whimsical ideas people have about what should be done with their earthly remnants. The main sticking point when it comes to making objects out of dead humans is often the nebulous idea of "desecration of a corpse." Because there is no consistent legal definition of what that phrase means, and some states' laws rely on community standards to draw the line on what we consider to be outside the bounds of those standards, corpse desecration is ultimately in the eye of the beholder.

Autopsies and cremation were viewed as desecration throughout the first century or so of American history, and those who committed these acts of desecration could be prosecuted by the state for criminal acts or found liable to the family of the deceased for civil damages.

In 2018, I read a newspaper article about an outfit called Save My Ink Forever that removed and preserved about 70 percent of a Canadian man's tattooed skin. I got in touch with Save My Ink Forever's Kyle Sherwood, a licensed funeral director and embalmer who had been working with Charles Hamm. In the three years since I'd met Hamm, the NAPSA nonprofit had folded. Sherwood and his father continued the work using a different business model, one that cultivates relationships with American funeral homes to arrange the skin's removal and preservation after someone dies. As a funeral director, he had seen an increase in customers looking for bespoke experiences surrounding their loved ones' and their own deaths. More and more people, living and dead, came into his funeral home sporting tattoos, which, as a tattooed person himself, he noticed. He echoed Hamm's sentiment that burying or cremating these works of art on skin would be a waste. "It'd be a shame for some of these wonderful pieces of art to never be seen again. It'd be like getting rid of the *Mona Lisa*."

I understood how he felt. While I was talking on the phone with Kyle Sherwood, my new tattoo was still healing on my forearm. I had decided to get a tattoo of an image combining a historical bookplate I found in some of the books I consulted during my many visits to the College of Physicians of

Philadelphia and an altered image of their Historical Medical Library logo. It features a butterfly atop a skull atop an old book and a banner with the Montaigne quote QUE SAIS-JE? ("What do I know?"). To me, it perfectly encapsulates the things I hold dearest in the world: nature, death positivity, lifelong learning, curiosity, and rare books. I found a woman tattoo artist who specializes in a woodcut look to create my tattoo and booked our appointment months in advance. Every choice was steeped in intention and incredibly personal and meaningful to me. As soon as it was finished, I texted a picture of my tattoo to Anna Dhody, my Anthropodermic Book Project teammate and the Mütter Museum's curator, who immediately proclaimed it "jar worthy"—the highest compliment, coming from her.

Given all this preservation talk, I couldn't help but think: What if I did have this tattoo preserved after my death and donated it to the Mütter? It would be in keeping with my love of the place and my feelings about the others whose bodies are there, too, though my choice would be made with full consent. Donating my body, or interesting parts of it, to the Mütter Museum would certainly be legal,* but I still had questions about the legality of indefinitely preserving human remains and the unusual methods one would use to preserve my jar-worthy tattoo. "We do a little bit better than a jar," Sherwood assured me.

Regarding the law, Sherwood holds a similar view to Hamm's. "Not liking it and it being a legal issue are two com-

---

* The Mütter Museum's FAQ states they accept body donations only in the rarest of circumstances, like the 2018 donation of a second skeleton with fibrodysplasia ossificans progressiva (FOP). In life Carol Orzel suffered from this incredibly rare and debilitating genetic disease where one's connective tissue turns into bone. She wished to donate her remains for research and display at the Mütter, where many living patients visit the remains of her fellow FOP sufferer Harry Eastlack. In the event that the museum has a curatorial interest in your remains, the preservation, preparation, and transport is on you.

pletely different things," Sherwood said, "and at this point, we've had enough exposure one way or another that if there was a legal issue someone would have come knocking on our door by now."

My friend Tanya Marsh, a legal professor at Wake Forest University who literally wrote the book on the laws regarding human remains in the United States (aptly titled *The Law of Human Remains*), is not so sure.

"If I had a [human] skull in my office in North Carolina, could they come after me?" said Marsh, referring to either a county prosecutor or state attorney general who would have jurisdiction over such matters. "They could absolutely come after me. Would they win? I don't know." Technically, Sherwood and Marsh agree, prosecuting desecration of a corpse is complaint-based, but Sherwood assumes that if Save My Ink Forever were on the wrong side of the law, someone would have tested them by now.

Why is the law so murky around what one can and cannot do with a corpse? The main issue is that, in legal terms—just like in the body-snatching days—a corpse is neither a person nor property. A dead body has no inherent rights, nor can a living person have true ownership over it.

The concept of the corpse as neither person nor property comes from the English common law and ecclesiastical law upon which U.S. laws are based. From the founding of the United States onward, U.S. and U.K. laws have diverged regarding human remains. In the United States, there is really only one federal law regarding human remains: the Native American Graves Protection and Repatriation Act (NAGPRA), which was enacted in 1990 after much lobbying from Native Americans to protect their ancestors' remains from being held in museums and sold as curiosities. Aside from NAGPRA, laws governing human remains are state-based, where even the definitions of what constitutes human remains are inconsistent, let alone what's permissible to do with them.

The U.S. legal system has developed what Marsh's book refers to as a "blazingly idiosyncratic" focus on the dying wishes of a person regarding their remains, which is absent from most other countries. That tendency would seem to favor enterprises like Save My Ink Forever, or an individual choosing to have a posthumous book made from her skin, but the legal risks associated with pushing these boundaries would be beyond the pale for most medical professionals or funeral directors carrying out the work on behalf of the deceased. Who would put their professional life on the line to be a guinea pig for testing these state laws? Passing legislation to allow or disallow practices such as preserving tattoos or binding books in human skin seems unlikely, as there would have to be a large constituency demanding such action from their representatives. As Tanya Marsh explained to me, "As a society we can either choose laws that reflect what we want to do and follow those laws, or we can choose to not really give a shit. And right now, we're kind of in a 'not really give a shit' world for a lot of this." She sighed. "It doesn't make me cynical at all."

Most of the other countries I've explored in my bibliophilic travels have more prescriptive laws around human remains, usually specifying how they should be kept in public institutions. Until the early twenty-first century, the national museums of England, Northern Ireland, and Wales (which, for simplicity's sake, I'll call "the U.K.," excluding Scotland, for reasons I'll get to later) had laws against the disposal of any objects from their collections, including human remains, which made repatriation claims difficult. More than sixty thousand human remains (from skeletons to anatomical wet specimens) are currently housed in U.K. museums, approximately 75 percent of them uncovered in the past few decades during land development excavations, so the majority won't be subject to repatriation efforts because they were local corpses. In the U.K. there's a legal distinction between human remains and an object made using human remains "through the application of skill," a distinction usually referring to tribal objects, but that would also apply to a human-skin-bound book. In this view, a skeleton is deemed human remains but an anthropodermic book would be considered a cultural artifact. This definition—absent from U.S. state and federal law—helps to illustrate the different thought processes at play with the Hunterian's decision to cremate William Corder's skeleton and give his ashes to a relative, and the Moyse's Hall Museum's denial of that same relative's request for Corder's purported skin-bound book and tanned scalp. In addition to the other reasons mentioned in this book for the museums' disparate decisions, in the eyes of the law these types of remains from the same person are viewed quite differently.

The U.K. law also makes distinctions regarding the age of the human remains when deciding what can or cannot be done with them. In the United States there are different rules regarding archaeological remains versus the freshly dead, with little guidance regarding the time in between. Most of the human remains in museums are between one hundred and three hundred years old, which corresponds with the historical period during which Europeans were stealing and buying human remains. Today, repatriation requests for remains from that time frame are the most successful. Tribes' claims to remains more than three hundred years old face a greater burden of proof.

The Human Tissue Act (HTA) of 2004 in the U.K. is very exacting compared to the nebulous American laws; it explicitly lists the tissues covered by the act. For example, skin is protected, but blood is not. Hair or nails from a living person are not covered, but hair or nails removed from a dead person are subject to the law. The line seems to be drawn at what can be regenerated biologically. The HTA requires that public institutions obtain both proof of consent and an often prohibitively expensive public display license for any bodies of people who died in the past hundred years. As all known cases of anthropodermic bibliopegy housed in the U.K. are more than a century old (though I can't help but wonder how the Wheatleys would be considered if they were across the pond), the U.K. libraries and museums don't need to meet these requirements, which works out well for them, because consent was almost never a factor in the creation of the objects in their possession. The age of the anthropodermic objects should also clear those seeking to buy or sell them on the antiquarian book market.

Scotland, home of the alleged William Burke skin book, has even more restrictive laws than the U.K. In addition to the U.K.'s restrictions, Scotland limits research on human remains less than one hundred years old. Under Scots law, items modified by human skill are also considered human remains. Scots law also prohibits the display of remains that were the result of anatomical examination, which you'd think would outlaw displaying the William Burke artifacts. But the Museum of the Royal College of Surgeons of Edinburgh and the Anatomical Museum at the University of Edinburgh were granted permanent exceptions to this rule, so William Burke's remains remain.

The Maori Toi moko, preserved tattooed heads taken from their homeland and added to the collections of many Western museums, are a good example of how different countries' museums deal with the same quandary. In 2007, the Field Museum in Chicago voluntarily repatriated their Maori remains, which were received by New Zealand's national museum, Te Papa. There was no law compelling them to do so, but the curators decided it was an ethical best practice to return the heads. Some smaller English museums repatriated their Toi moko, but officials at the British Museum argued that because the Toi moko were made by the application of skill, they were artifacts, not remains, and therefore not appropriate for repatriation.

Some small museums in Scotland also repatriated their Toi moko collections. When the mayor of Rouen attempted to send their museum's Toi moko back to New Zealand, the French ministry of culture blocked him from doing so, citing laws against removing works of art from museums. Later, France passed a law allowing museums to repatriate Toi moko specifically, but the patrimony laws regarding other human remains in French collections remain for now.

Despite France's reluctance to consider human remains for repatriation, the country's laws around the use of human bodies in other regards are strictest of all. Article 16 of the French Civil Code declares that the human body is inviolable and expressly prohibits many practices dealing with altering genetics, and even surrogacy. The penal code punishes perpetrators of "any attack on the integrity of the body, by any means whatsoever" with prison time and steep fines. For those considering doing any sales or innovative services regarding corpses, France is off the table. Charles Hamm saw great potential for

Save My Ink's services almost everywhere worldwide but France. People wishing to buy and sell skulls and skin books feel the chilling effects of the French laws, which is why I suspected, early on in my quest, that there were far more alleged French anthropodermic books than I'd ever find evidence of in public collections. After years of fits and starts, I would learn to trust my hunches.

{ 12 }

THE FRENCH CONNECTION

The Richelieu Library of the Bibliothèque nationale de France is nestled in the heart of Paris, in a building encircling the remnants of a seventeenth-century palace like a cocoon. The BnF's manuscript reading room is a long corridor with red walls and matching plush carpet that dampens sound in the already quiet room. The ceiling is gilded with painted pastoral scenes and a half dozen ostentatious chandeliers that speak to a palatial past before the modern addition of rows of plain-Jane wooden tables and chairs for researchers. In hushed tones, I fumbled my way through requesting three medieval Bibles rumored to be bound in human skin, the oldest by far that I would see in my research. The awe I feel when I'm holding a rare book increases with the length of time it had to travel to get to my hands; these books had seen countless sunrises and they were still here. I unwrapped the first book from its brown paper covering.

The style of handwriting on one of the first pages of this

Bible indicated that the note was added centuries after a monk copied out the thirteenth-century text. An eighteenth-century Sorbonne librarian, Antoine Augustin Lambert Gayet de Sansale, wrote that the book's binding was human: "sur peau humaine."

Sansale's note inside the next book translated as, "Abbot Rive alleged that this vellum was the skin of a woman. On the contrary I think it is the skin of an Irish stillborn lamb." An exceptional beauty, the book's binding was a deep burgundy and its pages were made from the smoothest, whitest parchment I had ever seen. They were so thin that they felt as though they defied physics; whichever monk created this Bible was truly a master of bookcraft.

The final Bible, known as a *décrétale*, had a shiny, malachite green binding that was cracking and splintering everywhere. The parchment inside, however, was so pristine that in spite of the eight hundred years since its creation, it was easy to distinguish the smooth side of the animal's hide versus the rougher side where hair once grew. Tiny pieces of the green leather fell on my desk and clothes as I gingerly leafed through the Bible. The thought crossed my mind that it was unlikely the BnF would ever submit these books to testing, and that I was currently wearing a few pieces of the binding that were plenty big enough to send to the lab. But stealing from the BnF would feel like pilfering from the collection plate. I made sure all the errant scraps of leather of undetermined origin were returned to the brown paper whence they came. Should the BnF ever agree to test these books of their own accord, and they turned out to be real human skin, I would be truly flabbergasted. These books are so old that it's impossible to trace their stories back past that Sorbonne librarian, Gayet de Sansale, scribbling the flyleaf notes. I hoped to uncover more of the other rumored French anthropodermic books, and was convinced my best choice was to go to Hell.

Hell, it appears, is in the François-Mitterrand location of the Bibliothèque nationale de France, and it couldn't be more different from my religious experience at their Richelieu location. It sits on a concrete vista that feels larger than anything else in Paris, with four imposing towers meant to evoke open books. Entering the building, I passed through more levels of security than I did in the Charles de Gaulle airport, then navigated endless Kafkaesque corridors until I finally found Room Y. Room Y houses the collection that the BnF refers to as *l'Enfer*, or Hell. *L'Enfer* is not just a cheeky nickname—the books in this room are marked with ENFER as their location. In the 1830s, *l'Enfer* was where the library separated their most salacious books, "contrary to good morals," from the rest of their collections. If I were going to find the legendary human-skin-bound copy of the Marquis de Sade stories *Justine et Juliette*, for example, Hell seemed like a smart place to look.

Unlike other trips, where I went only to see specific volumes, at the Mitterand I was grasping at straws—hoping that maybe one of these Sades would be *the* Sade, often mentioned in passing in writings about human skin books—but with no actionable leads to follow. I requested stacks of promising books pulled from the depths of Hell, including three Sades from the 1790s, and any book that had a title similar to ones I was seeking, but found no signs inside the books of possible anthropodermic bindings.

As the open hours of the BnF were dwindling, I left Hell for a more accessible area of the library, where I attempted a Hail Mary pass at a twentieth-century reference work about French bookbinding, not expecting much. Within the 1932 two-volume set, *La reliure française de 1900 à 1925* by Ernest de Crauzat, I found an article about books bound in human skin that recycled some of the same old French Revolution rumors that I had come across early in my research. What I didn't expect to find were about half a dozen photos of actual books that included tattooed skin as part of the binding. There was even a photo of *Éloge des seins* (In Praise of Breasts), with a human nipple smack in the middle of the cover. I was floored—never before had I seen any human skin books that were so obviously of human origin. The images were marked with captions denoting the books' locations in private collections, like "Bibliothèque R. Messimy," but little more detail.

That was when it dawned on me: Hell was not the best place to be searching for skin books. Any true anthropodermic books in France probably resided within old, moneyed private libraries, and the likelihood that some nosy American librarian was going to weasel her way into that world to get a peek at these controversial collections was slim to none. Seeing these photos shook my disbelief around some of the more outlandish French anthropodermic book tales. What of the rumors about Abbot Jacques Delille—dubbed "the French Virgil" and lauded by Voltaire before his sudden death at age thirty-four—whose skin was stolen from the mortuary table and used to bind books of his poetry? Or Verlaine's 1897 book of poetry, *Chair*, with a tattooed phallus on its front cover and a sword-pierced heart on its back cover? Crauzat, who clearly had the kind of access to French book collectors that I could only dream of, estimated that he knew of twenty-seven anthropodermic books in French collections, and that there were a lot more where they came from: "If we had the power, like Don Zombullo in *Diable boîteux*, to pass through walls and roofs and to slip surreptitiously into the homes of bibliophiles and rifle through their libraries, we would undoubtedly find more examples. But how many? We would certainly not reach fifty."

"Fifty? Imagine fifty," I gasped when I read that line. If there were anywhere close to fifty French human skin books, adding them would double the current known amount of even alleged anthropodermic books in the world to one hundred, as far as I had counted. But after seeing the images in Crauzat's book, I thought anything was plausible.

After my sad attempt at research at the BnF, I resigned myself to thinking that I would never gain access to the secret underground of French collectors of alleged human skin books. Imagine my surprise when they came to find me.

> When, at length, we had concluded our
> examination, and the intense excitement of the time had,
> in some measure, subsided, Legrand, who saw that I was
> dying with impatience for a solution of this most
> extraordinary riddle, entered into a full detail
> of all the circumstances connected with it.
>
> —EDGAR ALLAN POE, *The Gold-Bug*

WITH INCREASING REGULARITY, our team hears from private collectors with questions about testing books, but they rarely follow up with actual samples. While the Anthropodermic Book Project focuses on anthropodermic books held in public collections, the chemists on my team will often conduct tests for private collectors as well. We believe the tests could be useful for weeding out fakes in the private market, and any verified human skin book adds a lot to our understanding of the history of the practice. While the owners of occult books sometimes claim they own an anthropodermic book, we have yet to test an occult work that's turned out to be made from human skin. So when I heard from the French occult rare book seller Sébastien Vatinel of Les Portes Sombres, who had actually collected samples from a French grimoire called *Le triple vocabulaire infernal*—a manual focusing on witchcraft and demonology from about 1840—I was excited. I got downright giddy when he also included samples of two *more* books: a much older witchcraft book, *De l'imposture des diables* (1579) and an 1892 French edition of *Le scarabée d'or* (*The Gold-Bug*) by Edgar Allan Poe, both of which belonged to an avid occult book collector, Frédérick Coxe. When I asked Coxe if he could tell me more about his strange treasures, he wrote, "I stay at your entire disposal for any further informations." *Charmant!*

Coxe is in his midforties and runs his family's wine business in France. He has had a penchant for occult books since he was fifteen years old. "Those books make me dream," he wrote to me. "How incredible it was to discover that such books really exist. My purpose was very soon to become one of the greatest collectors of those marvelous pieces of an obscure history." An older occult collector by the name of Guy Bechtel took Coxe under his wing, advising him that it was better to buy one very beautiful book per year rather than twelve modest ones. Taking that advice, Coxe slowly built a collection of astoundingly rare occult texts; some of his necromantic volumes come from the very dawn of printing. The *De l'imposture des diables* that Coxe wanted us to test once belonged to his mentor Bechtel, which he did not know until he discovered notes inside the book in Bechtel's hand that noted the previous owner's "interesting but doubtful" assertion that it was bound in human skin.

Coxe bought the Poe book from a bookseller in San Francisco. Though he lives in France, Coxe was not worried about the legality of his books if they were determined to be human skin, because the witchcraft book was not sold as an anthropodermic book; he just suspected that it might be. The other was purchased in the United States, where the relatively recent age of the book and its potential status as human remains meant it was not expressly illegal to sell in some countries. Of course, he wanted both of them to be genuine. "If not, nevermind, it is a great adventure," he wrote. "I am like a little boy in front of his present, near the Christmas tree, waiting to open it."

For his part, Sébastien Vatinel was also hopeful for a positive result, which was unsurprising, because a real human skin book is instantly worth many times what the same book without such a binding could fetch. "Think about a book on demonology bound with human skin!" wrote Vatinel. "It will be almost a real *Necronomicon*!"

Vatinel's excitement came from more than just the thrill of the macabre. Before he became a rare book seller, he earned his Ph.D. in cellular biology and worked in proteomics, the scientific field of studying proteins, from which our PMF test derives. He knew our methods would work. He thinks PMF testing could help ease skepticism in the marketplace around these extraordinary books.

"The human skin books are always coming with an authenticity doubt," he wrote to me. "A French expert says that we can discriminate pork and human skin by counting the pores of the skin . . . I am very suspicious about that." Vatinel would like to convince other antiquarian booksellers of the benefits of adopting peptide mass fingerprinting tests in these cases.

He told me that if his alleged anthropodermic book turns out to be made of pigskin, he will lose money. And if it's human? "It's complicated!" Because of French laws, he couldn't really sell a book made out of human remains, and he has seen public auctions including such items canceled for this reason. He had been in talks with potential purchasers while he awaited our results.

One of his potential buyers was Madeleine Le Despencer. She is a London-based collector of antique books and objects relating to occultism, Catholicism, pornography, eroticism, and stage magic. She told me that a human skin book appeals to her as "delightfully rare and beautiful, the type of object that produces a frisson between its beauty and its transgressive qualities." She, too, was excited to hear from Vatinel regarding the final verdict of the peptide mass fingerprinting test, because the historical provenance and stories surrounding her books can mean as much as their contents. "In the case of an anthropodermic book, I would be happy to know the binding is indeed of human origin," Le Despencer explained. "However, if a book has been passed down centuries and treated with dread and reverence as if it were indeed a human skin binding, then I would be just as taken with the item, as it carries with it a lovely narrative and history. I might even hesitate to test such a book just to allow the mystery to remain."

I found these collectors and their bookish reverie beguiling. Besides book historians, there are few people in this increasingly digitally oriented world who appreciate the physicality and uniqueness of books as objects this way. Interacting with people with a similar orientation feels like entering into a special bond these days. We revere these books and admire their secrets, even as we strive to uncover them. But I wouldn't want to purchase my own anthropodermic book. Sure, I collect special and even rare books on my own champagne-taste-with-a-beer-budget level—I get my books signed whenever possible, I pick up the occasional Folio Society–style fancy modern edition, and I never buy paperbacks. Though I want to know all about anthropodermic books, and I think they have a wealth of information to offer, I don't intend to seek one for myself. The reason is not so much financial (though that would certainly be a barrier) as my prodding discomfort over owning human remains. Several of my friends own and even sell human remains, and it has taken me some time to determine where I stand on the subject. But I have a caveat: if someone donated an anthropodermic book to an institution where I worked, I would gladly care for it, and would see it as an opportunity to teach people about all of the ethical issues wrapped up in its existence. I feel I would be a better steward of such an object than most. As Vatinel alluded in his notes to me, our relationships with anthropodermic books are "complicated."

I FELT A KINSHIP with these collectors as we all waited with bated breath for the results. Luckily, our little cabal did not have to wait long.

I was at a Fourth of July barbecue and barn dance in Topanga Canyon when e-mails started to stream in from the French collectors. In front of a bunch of folk fans listening intently to a sweet child's ukulele rendition of "This Land Is Your Land," I loudly announced to a friend, "My French skin book test results are in!" To their credit, my friends are used to me by now.

In keeping with our previous findings regarding occult books, both of the witchcraft books turned out to be made from pigskin. As Sébastien Vatinel lamented, "The scientific truth takes from us a little piece of the dream, but that is the risky way of knowledge." For his part, Coxe was a little sad about his (still incredibly valuable and special) medieval grimoire, but enjoyed the adventure nonetheless, as he had predicted.

I can't say I was surprised at the occult books' results, though I did feel a little bad for the collectors. I had been mired so long in my historical research about anthropodermic bibliopegy, I had forgotten the joy of the anticipation and reward of getting the results and knowing just a tiny bit more about this strange world than anyone knew the day before. The events renewed my resolve to get more of the foreign books tested. The thrill of the hunt for knowledge restored, I'd find myself totally bowled over by the final revelation.

The brown spine of Edgar Allan Poe's *Le scarabée d'or* is adorned with a whimsical skull on a branch. Dangling from the skull is a gold bug on a string, precipitously hanging over a scythe and shovel. These elements might appear at first blush merely macabre, but they are all crucial to the plot of the book; it's not every day that one sees a book's bespoke binding double as a spoiler. A gilded stamp inside the cover reads "Relié en Peau Humaine," just like the handwritten notes in the BnF's medieval Bibles, but more intentionally included on the binding itself.

The Gold-Bug was Poe's big break, earning him a career-topping $100 in a newspaper contest, more than $3,300 today. The story is racially problematic by today's standards; Poe's attempt at writing in African American Vernacular English will make most modern readers fear they might cringe to death. But the book is important in that it popularized cryptography and even coined the term *cryptograph*. It is not as overtly goth as the ones that anchor Poe's legacy, but it has an air of mystery nonetheless. Charles Erskine Scott Wood, an anarchic Oregon frontier aristocrat who helped found the Portland Art Museum and make the Multnomah County Library free to the public, wrote an amazing inscription on the book's front endpapers:

> Dear John—What a tribute to the morbid death-loving Poe to find the "Gold Bug" in human skin—or is it an attempt at a pun? Poe humani en peau humaine. C.E.S.W.

Coxe believes that "John" might be Wood's close friend John Steinbeck. Did Steinbeck own a human skin book? The provenance possibilities are delicious. The combination of these details makes for an undeniably charming rare volume, so it is understandable that it attracted Coxe enough to bid on it in an auction from the San Francisco dealer PBA Galleries in 2016.

Now, our team has confirmed scientifically that the $850 he paid for a real human skin book was quite a steal. Just as the book's characters uncover a vast treasure after deciphering the code, our results matched the peptide mass fingerprints to their animals of origin.

Coxe has no plans to sell. "The purpose is to create one of the most interesting occult libraries," he explained. Perhaps at the end of his life or after his death, his Poe *en peau*, along with the other books of his dreams, will come up for sale once again. I wonder what the laws affecting human skin books will look like when that time comes.

In Coxe's Poe *en peau*, there is a bookplate with a skull and a snake sitting atop an open book bearing the name Russell van Arsdale Lee. A quick search turned up his 1982 obituary in

The New York Times. I was not surprised to discover that there was at least one doctor in the ownership lineage of this anthropodermic book. And quite a doctor he was: Dr. Russell Lee helped make group practice a common feature of American health care, and was a proponent for many controversial causes like abortion, free drugs for addicts, and prepaid national health insurance. Here's a sentence you don't see in many obituaries: "A leader in health education, Dr. Lee used $8,000 won in a poker game to help finance legislation to control venereal disease." He and his wife, Dorothy, had five children who all became doctors. When I got to their names, I gasped. "Wait, I *know* this family," I thought. One of his sons, Dr. Peter Lee, was a professor of medicine at my workplace, the University of Southern California. He was a beloved clinician and medical educator who helped establish Medicare. After he retired, he became an instructor in the Introduction to Clinical Medicine course that I occasionally help teach, and he developed the course of Professionalism and Practice of Medicine, which I consider an important foundation for our future doctors.

He organized an emeritus faculty book club, held at my library, until his death at age ninety-three, when his son donated many of his books to the library's collection. I was pretty new to my role of managing the collections at that time, and remember looking in awe over the shelves and shelves of books, trying to assess what we might want to add to the collection and what we might want to sell to support the library. His signature, lovingly penned into each book he owned, is emblazoned in my memory.

I remember so vividly a moment when my hand instinctively shot toward an otherwise unremarkable book by Ted Kennedy about health care policy. I don't know what it was, but my gut told me to open it, and inside was Ted Kennedy's inscription to Dr. Peter Lee, whom he had clearly worked with on policy matters. I wondered about the potential value of this kind of association copy—at that fleeting moment, under the administration of President Obama, it looked like true universal health care was just within reach. In fact, Dr. Lee's son, also named Peter, was a healthcare adviser in the Obama administration and became executive director for Covered California. We had to call this Peter Lee and offer the book to him. Giving the book back seemed the ethical thing to do, and it chilled me to think that I was the only person who could influence the future of this heirloom. I saved the book from ending up on our two-dollar book sale cart—or worse, in the dumpster—and sent it to the Lee family, where it belonged. How many personally or historically precious books meet the former fate every day? It was the first time that I felt the weight of my responsibility as a librarian, as a guardian of books.

To discover that the Poe *en peau*, this strange little anthropodermic book now nestled in a French occult library, has a legacy tracing back through the decades and across seas is a feeling that I'll never forget. As Coxe put it, this book made me dream. While some of its previous owners may remain forever in shadows, we now know that it has passed through the hands of the best and brightest in American medicine and perhaps literature as well—men whose work has affected all of our lives. And still there was this book, made using an unknown human's body. It is an object lesson in the history of medicine, bound in human skin.

HUMANE ANATOMY

L ibrarians are accustomed to fielding all sorts of questions, but few get asked about their corpse as often as I do. Even before I began researching anthropodermic books in earnest, my outspoken interests in death positivity and the history of sourcing bodies for anatomical learning led many to ask me what I wanted done with my own future corpse. Then in my twenties, I hadn't yet given the matter much thought. But around the time I started researching this book, I also began exploring the possibility of donating my body to a medical school.

The day after Memorial Day in 2014, I entered an auditorium on the University of Southern California's health sciences campus, where our first-year medical students were preparing for their own kind of remembrance. The students filled in the back half of the room, chattering over the tinkling piano as some older folks, more subdued, found their seats in the front. The two halves of the auditorium contained people with very different relationships to those being honored. They were all paying homage to the thirty body donors who were dissected by USC medical students that year. I was neither a medical student grappling with the realities of tearing apart a corpse for the sake of my education, nor a bereaved family member hoping to find some closure by learning about the good my loved one's choice had wrought. I was getting a rare sneak peek at what my future memorial might look like as a body donor. It probably says a lot about me that I had been looking forward to this ceremony for weeks.

Two emcees approached the podium. "Over one hundred and fifty hours and over two semesters, your loved ones have been our silent teachers," began a student named Benjamin Win, before welcoming Dr. Mikel Snow, director of USC's anatomy program, who explained the process that the donors' bodies go through to become viable learning tools. They were embalmed and then stored until classes started. Some were used for research, but the vast majority were used for teaching, with teams of students methodically working through the different body systems during their first year. These donors were the students' first patients, providing the lifelong seat of their understanding of the human body and instilling a profound awe that most of them will never forget.

The lights dimmed as a student played guitar and sang a song that he'd written, while others walked up the aisles with candles, one for each donor, and placed them on a table in the front. While this kind of ceremony could veer toward platitudes, real and rather complex emotions were shared among these strangers. A student named Warren Yamashita shared his poem, "Letter of Apology." He started out expressing his appreciation for the donor while making funny observations that resulted in peals of laughter from the audience, the kind of eruptive laughter you sometimes hear at funerals, when people are relieved to be permitted a moment of levity in a somber situation. Then Warren's poem took a sharp turn, and he choked up as he talked about the dissociative process necessary to perform dissections on a human corpse. He wished this donor would be the last patient whose humanity he would negate in order to do his job, but he knew he couldn't promise that. I was moved by the level of honesty the students displayed, even if it made some people uncomfortable. This was, after all, a very unusual circumstance in which to find ourselves. Some level of discomfort seemed not only appropriate but necessary.

I was glad that I went to see how contemporary students thank their body donors, because it is far more respectfully than I'd expected, given what I had come across in my history of medicine study. I couldn't imagine any of them jousting with body parts or taking trophies from corpses, as anatomy students did in bygone eras—let alone holding on to a piece of one of them to make into a book. I felt that after having worked with the donors all year, many of these budding physicians were likely just as curious about their lives as I was. Though some schools are now abandoning donor anonymity, the cadavers of the Keck School of Medicine of USC remained anonymous, so we weren't going to hear about why they made the unusual choice to donate. Since I am (as of this writing) still alive, I happily consent to tell the story of how I came to my decision.

The main impulse driving me to donate my body to our medical school was the thought that I was already spending my life educating medical students; it seemed fitting that I'd make use of my death in the same way. Yet I came to discover that the decision wasn't quite that simple. First, there was the matter of that pesky little "organ donor" box I checked when I got my California driver's license. You can't donate organs and also donate your entire body to scientific study; medical school cadavers can't arrive with parts missing. The requirements for whole body scientific donation can be very specific, but there is a much lower threshold to be a viable organ donor. You can be very young, very old, overweight, or die a traumatic death, and your organs can still save up to eight lives. Imagine saving eight people with what would otherwise just rot in the ground, and all the lives you would impact positively as a result of your act. Knowing that the list for patients needing an organ transplant in the United States has climbed to more than one hundred thousand people, with twenty dying each day for lack of replacement organs, it didn't feel right to hoard my organs after death.

The United States has an opt-in system, but if a family member objects to your donation, your organs won't be harvested. Would-be donors need to talk to their families about their wishes and just hope that, when faced with the decision, their families carry out their plans. So now I had a plan A: organ donation if I can be useful, with a side of plan B: donation of my full body to the medical school. My death was getting increasingly complicated, and I hadn't even started the paperwork!

The requirements for donating your body to a medical school vary from institution to institution, and they are often far stricter than the requirements for organ donation. At USC, you have to die from a noninfectious disease, and not from traumatic injuries like those sustained from a car accident or gunshot. You have to die within fifty miles of the campus, or your family has to pay to ship you there. You cannot exceed two hundred pounds at the time of death, as it makes it harder for students to move and flip your corpse, which they have to do often. Your body cannot come to the facility if you had a recent surgery before death, if you were autopsied, or if you have already been embalmed. You can't have signs of jaundice or decomposition, and your family has to notify the donor program within forty-eight hours of your death. Given all of these restrictions—in death as in life—most don't make the cut to get into medical school.

I figured I'd try my luck and apply anyway. If I'm neither a viable organ donor nor an eligible whole body donor, my plan C is boring old cremation, though I am now leaning toward aquamation, a more ecofriendly option that delivers similar results as cremation but uses water to process the remains instead of fire, and is now legal in California. My cremains, or aquamains or ashes or whatever you'd like to call them, would be scattered at a secret location that only my husband and I know. Plan C is clearly subject to change over time; there are elements of green burial that I also find very appealing, because if I don't have to be preserved for student use I would prefer that no one risk their health embalming me. Circumstances like a job change or moving cities could impact my death plan as well. Imagine if my family had waited until the last minute to have these discussions, or worse, avoided the conversation altogether, like most Americans do. With so many options and strong emotions involved, it is both totally understandable and completely unacceptable that we have become a society where people avoid this subject. This tension is what initially drew me to the nascent death-positive movement, and then to begin holding public events called Death Salons, where people could open up conversations around death and learn from experts edging us toward a healthier, more empowering relationship with our mortality.

BY 2017, my book research had taught me more about the historical tension between medical education and the corpses used in that education than I could ever have anticipated. I hadn't seen Dr. Mikel Snow in person since my visit to the body donor appreciation ceremony three years prior, and I was about to learn for myself how those students felt the first day they met their cadavers.

Snow led me up to his office to scrounge up a loaner white coat—that potent symbol of the medical profession and its great responsibility. I put on the loose coat embroidered with a Dr. Habib's name and placed my recorder and notebook in its pockets. We walked down to the basement and through a set of doors, where the overpowering smell of formaldehyde hit me in the face. This roomful of corpses was nothing like the cozy nineteenth-century wood and brass decor of the Mütter Museum; this was the low-ceilinged, fluorescently lit, twenty-first-century USC medical school anatomy lab that housed all thirty-eight of the cadavers being studied that semester.

Snow got me situated before returning to his students. I went back to the main cadaver room alone, formaldehyde burning my nostrils. Most of the cadavers were surrounded by small groups of students rapidly quizzing one another, and the cacophony was as all-encompassing as the smell. A student marched up to me and asked a question, and I assured her I was the worst person to ask, despite my imposter white coat. I was here with my own questions, and she allowed me to sidle up to her group to observe as they reviewed for their exam on the thoracic cavity.

The students alternated between picking up organs such as a heart or lung, looking at the structures left behind by what they took away, consulting the *Netter's Atlas of Anatomy* on a music stand next to the cadaver, and conferring with an articulated fake skeleton, moving deftly among all these different learning tools while consulting with one another. Sometimes a student would rest the *Atlas* on the cadaver, leaving little pink smudge marks of viscera on the book. I couldn't help but think of Dr. Joseph Leidy and his *Elementary Treatise on Human Anatomy*, checking his book's proofs next to an open cadaver. The students were respectful of the body donor and also seemed at ease with his corpse. I noticed small twinges of discomfort on their faces only when it came time to lift and flip him. They took the lung that was sitting on his chest and put it back inside, followed by his heart, then put the cut-out rib section back on top like a puzzle piece locking into place. They wrapped him in a sheet, then again in plastic, then all six of them flipped him over. As I walked around the room, I caught glimpses of an earlobe here or there, but for the most part, the faces of the cadavers were covered with formerly white sheets, now tinged pink with blood. I felt like my eyes were bugging out of my head and I was swaying from the fumes. In contrast to my demeanor in pretty much every other situation, I was silent. This could be my cadaver one day, if I willed it so.

Back at my table, one of the women was saying she wanted to check out a female cadaver because she was interested in the structures of breast tissue. A bearded young doctor nodded to us from across the room, and the group enthusiastically flagged him down. The students lit up at his presence, and it was instantly clear that the man loved his job and his students loved him in return. He glanced down at my white coat only to see his own name emblazoned on my chest, but to his credit, he didn't make a big deal of it. I flushed with embarrassment as the real Dr. Michael Habib showed the curious student the breast tissue in the anatomy book. It was no small feat to focus my attention on the illustration of the breast's inner workings the very week I was weaning my baby—as if my own body wasn't already feeling a little too conspicuous around this cohort of corpses.

Habib was peppered with questions from the students, who punctuated his responses with enthusiastic exclamations of "Yeah!" and "Cool!" One well-answered question elicited a group high five, and Habib quipped, "People always ask about medical students doing drugs like cocaine. But I'm like, why would I do drugs when I can just be *right*?" I totally got why they loved Dr. Habib. He had just been on my friend Alie Ward's science podcast, *Ologies*, and it turned out his USC anatomy assistant professorship is only a part-time gig—he spends the rest of his time as a research associate in the Dinosaur Institute at the Natural History Museum of Los Angeles County. "You get a big cup of coffee in the morning, you take apart a human being. So that's my deal for about half the time," he told Ward. "The other half of the time I go and play with dinosaurs."

I couldn't believe it. Right here at my own institution there was a twenty-first-century Joseph Leidy—a skilled anatomist and paleontologist—but with a sense of humor and hopefully no penchant for purloining human skin to bind books.*

I was feeling increasingly light-headed and the students

---

* Later, Dr. Habib would tell me he is what they call an academic descendant of Joseph Leidy—meaning if you follow the lineage from Dr. Habib up through his academic adviser and that person's advisers and so on, eventually you hit Dr. Joseph Leidy. It's a small professional world after all.

were still going strong in their exam review. I left, feeling strange, like I had been thrust back into a newly unfamiliar above-ground world from an underground one where the rules of engagement were totally different. Being up close to an open corpse for the first time, and imagining myself being flipped over and bits of me handled and moved around, made me think of my body donation decision in a different light. Far from scaring me off, it was clear now how useful this experience was to the medical students, and the obvious worth of that donation overrides any residual squeamishness on my part. Just weeks into their first semester, the students had already lost a lot of their trepidation around their cadavers; I had no doubt that an entire year of this exposure must have a huge emotional and psychological impact on them.

I caught up with one of the students in my group to get her impressions on that transformation. Alodia Girma said the idea of her becoming a doctor had been nurtured by her Ethiopian immigrant parents as far back as she could remember. Then, the great care she received at seventeen during her own spinal fusion surgery and recovery sealed the deal for her. As an undergraduate, she worked as a scrub in an emergency room, which was the first time in her life that she saw a dead body. When she began medical school, she recognized that the bulk of her peers had never seen a dead body at all before that moment, not even at a funeral. But viewing a body wasn't nearly the same as cutting one open. Her first day at the lab, she kept telling herself, "Yes, this is a person, but you need to do this." After her second or third day, she felt right at home.

Meanwhile, in her Professionalism in the Practice of Medicine course (the same class that Dr. Peter Lee—whose father owned the anthropodermic Poe book—helped create), Girma had been spending a lot of time learning how to speak with the dying and their families. The students worked with an actor portraying a dying patient so they could practice maintaining empathy while explaining palliative care and hospice options. Girma said the experience helped shift her assumption that physicians were supposed to avoid death—including talking about it—at all costs. "I think we talked about it more than I ever expected we would talk about it this soon in our medical career," Girma said of her death and dying training, "but I think it's making us more holistic physicians who actually empathize with our patients more." That was music to my death-positive medical librarian ears.

Everyone wants empathy from their doctors, but the medical profession can't agree on what that really means. In a 2018 *Academic Medicine* commentary, the clinical psychologist Anne Dohrenwend attempted a working definition, first pointing out that empathy is not sympathy (a physician expressing her feelings of concern for a patient), nor is it "putting oneself in another's shoes," an impossibility especially across the huge cultural, class, and social gaps often present between doctors and patients. Some call this "cognitive empathy," where the doctor attempts to think about patients' feelings without actually feeling the emotions themselves, because to do so would render them unable to function.

"Empathy is a conscious, strenuous, mental effort to clarify a patient's muddy expression of her experience using a soft interpretation of her story," Dohrenwend wrote. "Employing the empathic process involves the distilling or connecting of feelings and meanings that are associated with a patient's experience while simultaneously identifying, isolating, and withholding one's own reactions to that patient and her experience." The empathetic doctor must think "as if" she inhabits the patient's world during the clinical encounter, without losing sight of the fact that her own natural reactions would likely be very different from her patient's. The doctor must strive to clarify the patient's "*almost* articulated fear," accept where the patient is in his journey even if the doctor thinks he's headed in the wrong direction, and take the time to think and reflect about this loaded interaction. Some refer to the special kind of empathy necessary in the doctor-patient relationship as clinical empathy. In the physically and emotionally taxing environment of the clinic, empathy is a lot to ask of a doctor. But a lack of empathy can cause irreparable harm to both the doctor and the patient.

Patients with empathetic doctors are more likely to participate positively in their own health care, taking healthful actions such as adhering to prescribed drug regimens. Diabetics with empathetic doctors, for example, are more successful in keeping cholesterol and blood sugar levels in check. The open communication facilitated by a skilled, empathetic physician improves the quality and detail of the information the patient provides to the doctor, allowing them to better diagnose and treat ailments. Better communication also decreases malpractice lawsuits, a desirable result for all clinicians and hospitals. Investing in empathetic doctors is not just a nice ideal, it makes financial and legal sense for the hospital.

The gold standard of measuring clinician empathy is the Jefferson Scale of Physician Empathy (JSPE). Since its development in 2001, it has been translated into fifteen languages and the result patterns are similar worldwide. The questionnaire includes statements about approaches to patient interactions but also about interest in literature and art, based on theories that tie those personal interests to an increased understanding of pain and suffering. A sense of humor also improves the doctor-patient relationship and is considered in the JSPE. I suspect Dr. Habib scores highly on this test.

The student-specific version of the JSPE routinely finds that medical students like those in my anatomy lab group start their educations with a relatively normal or high degree of empathy, but their empathy drops precipitously during their third year, when they actually start interacting with real live patients. This tendency is dangerous for a number of reasons, not only because it means patients are interacting with burned-out, apathetic medical students whom they perceive as full-fledged doctors, but also because the behaviors students develop early on could prove difficult to shake going forward. Why does empathy so often get lost in the chaotic shuffle of the hospital?

I believe the answer lies in the inhumane expectations for medical students and doctors. Early career physicians report the lowest satisfaction levels with their career choice, the highest incidence of conflict between their work and home lives, and the strongest feelings of depersonalization. In the face of stress and exhaustion, young doctors cope by turning their patients into more manageable objects. It's this mindset that could eventually have led doctors in the past to dehumanizing abuses like creating anthropodermic books. Though the abuses of depersonalization might look different today than when these books were made, the detrimental effects of the clinical gaze on patients endure.

When thinking about anthropodermic books, we can't simply fault the doctors of the past for engaging in behavior that was tacitly or explicitly sanctioned by the laws and mores of their time and place in history; nor can we expect them to retroactively adhere to the deeply important beliefs we now have about informed consent. The practice was never truly commonplace, but countless people—other doctors, book collectors, bookbinders, collectors' families, and newspaper reporters, just to name a few—turned a blind eye to what we would now see as an abhorrent affront to common decency. What we can do, and have a moral obligation to do, is examine the institutions in which these injustices were able to proceed, learn from their mistakes, and critically view the pernicious ways these mindsets might persist in our current society and fight to eradicate them. We need to prevent the Dr. Habibs and future Dr. Girmas of the world from allowing their curiosity and compassion to be stripped away, sending them down the well-trodden path of depersonalization that enabled the Dr. Joseph Leidys of history to strip humanity from their patients as well.

OF ALL THE INCREDIBLE but ethically questionable specimens that Leidy contributed to the Mütter Museum, I think about one most of all. Set between the skeletons of a dwarf and a person of average height, the Mütter American Giant towers over his case-mates at seven feet, six inches tall—the tallest skeleton on display in North America. His spine is curved, his rib cage sharply distended.

Nobody knows who this man was. Some armchair sleuths have attempted to figure out his identity, but the historical record provides little more than this: his body appeared in 1877 on an auctioneer's slab in Kentucky and was sold to Leidy on the condition that he ask no questions about the body's origins. For all Leidy knew, this man might have been stolen from the grave by body snatchers, or worse. Leidy bought him anyway.

In life, this man suffered from an excess of human growth

hormone (HGH), produced by his brain's pituitary gland. When it develops in childhood, this condition is called gigantism—think André the Giant. Although the disease is rare, the visual symptoms make it a fairly easy one to diagnose. When HGH overproduction occurs in adults—people whose growth plates are already fused—the disease is called acromegaly. Usually caused by benign brain tumors that form around the patient's pituitary gland, acromegaly produces a constellation of symptoms that are subtle, varied, and often misinterpreted. Patients can suffer for years, eventually dying of complications caused by enlarged organs and the resultant added stress on the body's systems before their doctors see the forest for the trees.

Whenever I visit the Mütter, I always stop to give a respectful nod to the Mütter American Giant. He reminds me of my mom. When I was a young girl, my mother started getting headaches. She started to complain about a lot of ailments that she never had before: her joints hurt; she was often dizzy; her headaches made her vision blur to the point that her glasses became useless. When she visited her doctor, he prescribed drugs for each of her symptoms, one at a time, and sent her on her way. As she started going in more and more frequently, the receptionists began rolling their eyes. "Oh, it's you again," they said, sighing.

Mom was mortified by the idea that people thought she was a hypochondriac. Over time, she started to believe that maybe they were right. Coming from a working-class Irish Catholic background, she had been taught to respect people in positions of authority. When police, clergy, or doctors spoke, she was supposed to sit there, listen, and do what she was told. So that's what she did—for years.

Her health continued to deteriorate. More strange symptoms emerged. She gained weight and wasn't able to lose it. Her rings no longer fit on her swollen fingers. Slowly, the shape of her face began to change—her brow and jawline protruded, erasing her once delicate features. Her feet grew by a few shoe sizes. She even swore that she grew a couple of inches in height. She tried to keep her bizarre health complaints to herself, except when her symptoms were unbearable. Even then, she felt ashamed of reporting them. Years elapsed before Mom's gynecologist (of all people!) took the unusual step of ordering an MRI of her brain. The test revealed that she had acromegaly.

Luckily, my mother was diagnosed in time to have brain surgery to remove her tumors. If she had been left untreated much longer, she could have died from severe complications. Not that surgery was a completely safe option, and my mom knew this. I was thirteen when she took the opportunity to change her kids' last names to match our father's, thinking it would ease matters for us should she never check out of the hospital. "Oh my god, I was so scared," she told me later. "I just cried—all night, all the way there, the whole time—I just couldn't stop crying."

Because my mom's surgery was performed so late, her hormones couldn't return to normal levels on their own. To this day, her medication bottles nearly fill a tote bag. She injects synthetic HGH, which is derived from human cadavers and is sent to her home in a refrigerated bag. The side effects—and the costs—are crippling.

When I stand in front of the Mütter American Giant, I think about the rare hormonal imbalance that he and my mother have in common. I wonder if his doctor thought he was crazy, too—if he even had a doctor. I wonder whether he had a daughter like me who worried about him. I wonder what his name was, and I wonder whether the doctors who put him in a glass case more than 150 years ago ever considered these things. Did they see his skeleton as the remains of a person, or simply as a tool to teach medical students about a rare disorder?

Every time I see him, I feel pity and empathy for the life and death I presume he endured, even though I know it's all just the speculation of a twenty-first-century woman disconnected from his reality. Of all the complicated feelings I experience as I stand in front of his glass case, the strongest is gratitude for all that his presence in the museum has taught and continues to teach me.

When I hosted a Death Salon at the Mütter Museum in 2015, it felt like a homecoming in every way. Friends from all different areas of my life were present—my dearest friend since middle school took the event photos; a friend from high school checked people in; my friends' band played murder ballads. If I weren't so cognizant of my mortality, I'd have sworn it was my own funeral.

Although we lived only a brief drive away from the Philadelphia city limits when I was growing up, my mother almost never ventured into the city. It meant a lot to me that she gathered up the gumption to take a train into town all alone to experience my Death Salon event for herself. I had no idea how she would take all of it. She is pretty squeamish and on the superstitious side. I had good reason to fear that she would pass out, which, the staff tells me, is a common enough occurrence at the Mütter. But there was someone I really wanted my mother to meet.

Standing in front of the Mütter American Giant, Mom gamely read all the labels and nodded in approval. "I think everything they have on display here is great, because you can learn something from it or relate it to a person," she later reflected on the experience. Seeing him did bring back some memories of her frightening surgery.

"Imagine yourself going in for brain surgery," she said to me. "Did the doctor have a good night last night? Could you put your life in the hands of somebody that you don't even know?"

Millions of people have to make that leap of faith every day. We need to strive for the kind of humane health care that the Mütter American Giant, Mary Lynch, and Mom would all appreciate.

THE ANTHROPODERMIC BOOK PROJECT'S LIST OF CONFIRMED HUMAN SKIN BOOKS AS OF MARCH 2020

BIBLIOTHÈQUE ROYALE DE BELGIQUE

Félix Vicq-d'Azyr, *Essai sur les lieux et les dangers des sépultures.*

BOSTON ATHENÆUM

George Walton, *Narrative of the Life of James Allen, Alias George Walton, Alias Jonas Pierce, Alias James H. York, Alias Burley Grove the Highwayman . . .*

BROWN UNIVERSITY

Adolphe Belot, *Mademoiselle Giraud, My Wife.*
Hans Holbein, *The Dance of Death* (1816 edition).
Hans Holbein, *The Dance of Death* (1898 edition).
Andreas Vesalius, *Andreae Vesalii Bruxellensis . . . De humani corporis fabrica . . .*

CINCINNATI PUBLIC LIBRARY

Phillis Wheatley, *Poems on Various Subjects, Religious and Moral.*

COLLEGE OF PHYSICIANS OF PHILADELPHIA

Louis Barles, *Le nouvelles decouvertes sur toutes les parties principales de l'homme et de la femme.*
Louise Bourgeois, *Recueil des secrets de Louyse Bourgeois.*
Robert Couper, *Speculations on the Mode and Appearances of Impregnation in the Human Female.*
Charles Drelincourt, *De conceptione adversaria.*
Joseph Leidy, *An Elementary Treatise on Human Anatomy.*

THE GROLIER CLUB

Anonymous, *Le traicté de Peyne: poëme allégorique dédié à Monseigneur et à Madame de Lorraynne.*

HARVARD UNIVERSITY

Arsène Houssaye, *Des destinées de l'ame.*

THE HUNTINGTON LIBRARY, ART MUSEUM, AND BOTANICAL GARDENS

M.N. (Thomas Gibson), *Anatomy Epitomized and Illustrated.* . . .

UNIVERSITY OF CINCINNATI

Phillis Wheatley, *Poems on Various Subjects, Religious and Moral.*

UNIVERSITY OF PENNSYLVANIA

Bibliothèque nationale (de France), *Catalog des sciences médicales.*

NOTES

PROLOGUE: UNDER GLASS

4 *"most cherished possession"*: Helen Carter Leidy, letter to Dr. Packard, January 2, 1933. Historical Medical Library of the College of Physicians of Philadelphia.

6 *120 acres of manicured greenery*: The Huntington, "The Huntington Botanical Gardens," accessed November 18, 2019, https://www.huntington.org/gardens.

6 *eleven million items*: The Huntington, "Library Collections," accessed November 18, 2019, https://www.huntington.org/library-collections.

9 *identified only about fifty alleged anthropodermic books*: The Anthropodermic Book Project, "The Anthropodermic Book Project," accessed November 18, 2019, https://anthropodermicbooks.org.

10 *believe was Thomas Gibson*: The Huntington, catalog record for *Anatomy Epitomized and Illustrated . . .*, accessed November 18, 2019, http://catalog.huntington.org/record=b1767846.

10 *Originally published in 1682*: Victor Cornelius Medvei, *A History of Endocrinology* (Lancaster, England: MTP Press Limited, 1982), 140.

10 *previously owned by Dr. Blake Watson*: The Huntington, catalog record for *Anatomy Epitomized and Illustrated. . . .*

10 *former obstetrics department chair*: Blake H. Watson, "Specialist-General Practitioner Cooperation in an Obstetrical Department." *California Medicine* 75, no. 4 (October 1951): 307.

10 *This library*: Robert J. Moes, preface to *Thirty Books in the Library of the Los Angeles County Medical Association: A Compendium of Medical History* (Los Angeles: Friends of the LACMA Library, 1984), 11–12.

11 *"This is the skin of a White Man"*: The Huntington, catalog record for "Luke Swaatland Note on Skin, After 1779," accessed November 18, 2019, http://catalog.huntington.org/record=b1796511.

12 *"The Indians were remarkably kind"*: Edward Merrifield, *The Story of the Captivity and Rescue from the Indians of Luke Swetland: An Early Settler of the Wyoming Valley and a Soldier of the American Revolution* (Scranton, PA: 1915), 51.

12 *"To them it at first"*: Merrifield, *Luke Swetland*, 11.

12 *Many credit Noah Webster*: Florian Coulmas, *Guardians of Language: Twenty Voices Through History* (Oxford, U.K.: Oxford University Press, 2016), 120.

13 *The process goes like this*: Daniel P. Kirby et al., "Identification of Collagen-Based Materials in Cultural Heritage," *Analyst* 138 (2013): 4850.

13 *The MALDI plate*: Timothy P. Cleland and Elena R. Schroeter, "A Comparison of Common Mass Spectrometry Approaches for Paleoproteomics," *Journal of Proteome Research* 17 (2018): 938–39.

13 *Each animal family*: Michael Buckley et al., "Species Identification by Analysis of Bone Collagen Using Matrix-Assisted Laser Desorption/Ionisation Time-of-Flight Mass Spectrometry," *Rapid Communications in Mass Spectrometry* 23 (2009): 3852–53.

13 *explained to me*: Daniel Kirby, e-mail to the author, October 19, 2019.

13 *Bovidae family*: Mike Buckley et al., "Distinguishing Between Archaeological Sheep and Goat Bones Using a Single Collagen Peptide," *Journal of Archaeological Science* 37 (2010): 13.

14 *other members of the Hominidae family*: Samantha Brown et al., "Identification of a New Hominin Bone from Denisova Cave, Siberia Using Collagen Fingerprinting and Mitochondrial DNA Analysis," *Scientific Reports* 6 (2016): 2.

14 *Collagen... lasts far longer*: Sarah Fiddyment et al., "So You Want to Do Biocodicology? A Field Guide to the Biological Analysis of Parchment," *Heritage Science* 7, no. 35 (2019): 3.

14 *destroy much of the testable DNA*: Mim A. Bower et al., "The Potential for Extraction and Exploitation of DNA from Parchment: A Review of the Opportunities and Hurdles," *Journal of the Institute of Conservation* 33, no. 1 (2010): 5–6.

14 *can contaminate a sample*: Joachim Burger et al., "Palaeogenetics and Cultural Heritage. Species Determination and STR-Genotyping from Ancient DNA in Art and Artefacts," *Thermochimica Acta* 365 (2000): 143.

14 *Advances in historical and ancient DNA extraction*: M. D. Teasdale et al., "Paging Through History: Parchment as a Reservoir of Ancient DNA for Next Generation Sequencing," *Philosophical Transactions B* 370 (2015): 2.

14 *a new field called biocodicology*: Beasts2Craft, "Biocodicology: The Parchment Record and the Biology of the Book," accessed November 18, 2019, https://sites .google.com/palaeome.org/ercb2c/get-involved/workshops/folger.

14 *animal husbandry practices*: Niall J. O'Sullivan et al., "A Whole Mitochondria Analysis of the Tyrolean Iceman's Leather Provides Insights into the Animal Sources of Copper Age Clothing," *Scientific Reports* 6 (2016): 1–2.

14 *evidence of plague*: Alfonsina D'Amato et al., "Of Mice and Men: Traces of Life in the Death Registries of the 1630 Plague in Milano," *Journal of Proteomics* 180 (2018): 128.

15 *DNA in parchment*: Bower et al., "DNA from Parchment," 5–6.

15 *strict policies regarding destructive sampling*: Fiddyment et al., "So You Want to Do Biocodicology?"

15 *pioneering less destructive methods*: Sarah Fiddyment et al., "Animal Origin of 13th-Century Uterine Vellum Revealed Using Noninvasive Peptide Fingerprinting," *PNAS* 112 (2015): 15067–68.

15 *methods that are the least invasive*: Anita Quye and Matija Strlič, "Icon Heritage Science Group Ethical Sampling Guidance," The Institute of Conservation (ICON), January 2019, accessed November 18, 2019, https://icon.org.uk/system /files/documents/icon_hsg_ethical_sampling_guidance_-_jan_2019.pdf.

15 *next-gen DNA sequencing methods also cost more*: Fiddyment et al., "So You Want to Do Biocodicology?"

15 *biological sex*: Matthew Teasdale et al., "The York Gospels: A 1000-Year Biological Palimpsest," *Royal Society Open Science* 4 (2017): 8.

16 Anatomy Epitomized and Illustrated... *was bound in real human skin*: The Huntington, catalog record for *Anatomy Epitomized and Illustrated*....

16 *Swaatland note was written on cowhide*: The Huntington, catalog record for "Luke Swaatland."

16 *a truly American genre*: Gordon M. Sayre, "Slave Narrative and Captivity Narrative: American Genres," in *A Companion to American Literature and Culture*, ed. Paul Lauter (Malden: Wiley-Blackwell, 2010), 188.

16 *half of the objects we've tested so far have been made out of real human skin*: The Anthropodermic Book Project, "The Anthropodermic Book Project," accessed November 18, 2019, https://anthropodermicbooks.org.

17 *creepypasta*: Creepypasta Wiki, "What Is Creepypasta?," accessed November 18, 2019, https://creepypasta.fandom.com/wiki/Creepypasta_Wiki:What _Is_Creepypasta%3F.

1. THE FIRST PRINTING

20 *"I dedicate this book"*: "Je vous dédie ce livre, / à vous / qui avez été l'âme de la maison, / qui m'appelez dans la maison de dieu, / qui êtes partie avant moi / pour me faire aimer le chemin de la mort, / vous dont le souvenir est doux / comme le parfum des rives regrettées, / vous qui avez mis des enfants dans la maison, / vous qui ne reviendrez pas / mais qui avez toujours votre place au foyer, / vous qui avez été / la muse, la femme et la mère, / avec les trois beautés / la grâce, l'amour et la vertu; / à vous / que j'ai aimée, que j'aime et que j'aimerai." Translation by the author. Arsène Houssaye, *Des destinées de l'ame* (Paris: Calmann Lévy, 188-), Harvard Library, http://id.lib.harvard.edu/aleph/005786452 /catalog/.

21 *"If you look"*: "En le regardant attentivement on distingue facilement les pores de la peau. Un livre sur l'Ame humaine méritait bien qu'on lui donnait un vêtement humain..." Translation by the author. Houssaye, *Destinées de l'ame*.

21 *Wearing gloves*: The National Trust, "Why Wearing Gloves Puts Books at Risk," accessed November 19, 2019, https://www.nationaltrust.org.uk/features/why -wearing-gloves-puts-books-at-risk.

22 *high-powered microscopes*: Jacob Gordon, "In the Flesh? Anthropodermic Bibliopegy Verification and Its Implications," *RBM: A Journal of Rare Books, Manuscripts, and Cultural Heritage* 17, no. 2 (2016): 121.

22 *follicle patterns can be unreliable*: Fiddyment et al., "So You Want to Do Biocodicology?"

22 *Des destinées de l'ame was determined to be genuine*: Heather Cole, "The Science of Anthropodermic Binding," *Houghton Library Blog*, June 4, 2014, http://blogs .law.harvard.edu/houghton/2014/06/04/caveat-lecter/.

24 *"The analyses done here"*: Jack Eckert, e-mail to the author, April 2015.

25 *"Ovid's Metamorphoses"*: Jack Eckert, interview with the author, April 9, 2015.

26 *before books became mechanically produced*: David H. Tucker et al., "History of Publishing," in *Encylopædia Britannica*, updated March 8, 2018, https://www .britannica.com/topic/publishing/.

26 *Rebinding was especially popular*: David Pearson, *Provenance Research in Book History: A Handbook* (New Castle, DE: Oak Knoll Press, 2019), 172.

26 *"The latest upheavals"*: Jack Eckert, interview with the author, April 9, 2015.

27 *"This book should be buried"*: Comments on Heather Cole, "The Science of Anthropodermic Binding," *Houghton Library Blog*, June 4, 2014, http://blogs .law.harvard.edu/houghton/2014/06/04/caveat-lecter/.

27 *"Caveat Lecter"*: The post was later retitled with the less playful and more descriptive "The Science of Anthropodermic Binding."

27 *"Good news"*: Cole, "Science of Anthropodermic Binding."

27 *"shocking in its crudity"*: Paul Needham, "A Binding of Human Skin in the Houghton Library: A Recommendation," June 25, 2014, accessed March 7, 2015, http://www.princeton.edu/~needham/Bouland.pdf.

28 *"Although preservation"*: Needham, "A Binding of Human Skin."

28 *"A reader"*: Needham, "A Binding of Human Skin."

29 *"I really don't want"*: Daniel Kirby, interview with the author, April 9, 2015.

29 Using well-established techniques: Daniel Kirby, interview with the author, April 9, 2015.

29 a nineteenth-century Yup'ik: Kirby et al., "Identification of Collagen-Based Materials," 4856–57.

30 Alan Puglia: Daniel Kirby, interview with the author, April 9, 2015.

30 *"I've taught"*: Daniel Kirby, interview with the author, April 9, 2015.

31 a private database: Special thanks to Rebecca Michelson for her assistance in identifying an appropriate system and populating our database.

32 *"The modern consensus"*: Joseph L. Graves, "Race [does not equal] DNA: If Race Is a Social Construct, What's Up with DNA Ancestry Testing?," accessed November 5, 2019, http://www.tolerance.org/sites/default/files/general/Race%20does%20not%20equal%20DNA%20-%20TT50.pdf.

32 Bibliotheca politica: Jacob Gordon and Richard Hark, "Rumored Example of Anthropodermic Bibliopegy at Juniata College," *The Anthropodermic Book Project* (blog), November 17, 2015, https://anthropodermicbooks.org/2015/11/17/rumored-example-of-anthropodermic-bibliopegy-at-juniata-college/.

2. THIS DREADFUL WORKSHOP

36 Mark Twain Project: The Mark Twain Project, "Mark Twain Papers & Project: A Brief History," accessed August 13, 2018, http://www.marktwainproject.org/about_projecthistory.shtml.

36 the largest papyrus collection: The Bancroft Library, "About the Tebtunis Collection," accessed August 13, 2018, http://www.lib.berkeley.edu/libraries/bancroft-library/tebtunis-papyri/about-tebtunis-collection/.

37 Inside the book: L'office de l'église en François (Paris: Chez Pierre Le Petit, 1671), UC Berkeley Library, http://oskicat.berkeley.edu/record=b10357222~S6.

38 Republican generals: Gaston Variot, "Remarques sur l'autopsie et la conformation organique du supplicié Pranzini et sur le tannage de la peau humaine," *Bulletins et mémoires de la société d'anthropologie de Paris*, Seventh Series, 10 (1929): 45–46.

39 The Abbot of Montgaillard: Henri Clouzeau, "Les tanneries de peaux humaines aux châteaux de Meudon durant la période révolutionnaire: pour ou contre?," *Bulletin de l'association «Les Amis de Meudon»* 260 (2015): 19.

39 *"People tanned"*: "On tannait, à Meudon, la peau humaine, et il est sorti de cet affreux atelier des peaux parfaitement préparées; le duc d'Orléans, Égalité, avait un pantalon de peau humaine. Les bons et beaux cadavres de suppliciés étaient écorchés, et leur peau tannée avec un soin particulier. La peau des hommes avait une consistance et un degré de bonté supérieurs à la peau des chamois; celles des femmes présentait moins de solidité, à raison de la mollesse du tissu." Translation

by the author. L'Abbé de Montgaillard, *Histoire de France, depuis la fin du règne de Louis XVI jusqu'à l'année 1825, tome quatrième* (Paris: Moutardier, 1827), 290, https://gallica.bnf.fr/ark:/12148/bpt6k30607368.

39 *"read with the utmost caution"*: Hugh Chisholm, ed., "Montgaillard, Jean Gabriel Maurice Roques, Comte de," *Encyclopædia Britannica*, 11th ed. 18 (New York: Cambridge University Press: 1911): 782.

39 *Some moderate newspapers*: Clouzeau, "Les tanneries," 23–24.

39 *"Few histories"*: Lawrence S. Thompson, "Tanned Human Skin," *Bulletin of the Medical Library Association* 34, no. 2 (1946): 94

40 *last acts of the Committee of Public Health*: Clouzeau, "Les tanneries," 20–22.

40 *most credible chroniclers*: Lawrence S. Thompson, *Bibliologica Comica: Or Humorous Aspects of the Caparisoning and Conservation of Books* (Hamden, CT: Archon Books, 1968), 129–30; Clouzeau, "Les tanneries," 19.

40 *Renaissance-era townhouses*: Musée Carnavalet, "Museum Carnavalet," accessed November 8, 2017, http://www.carnavalet.paris.fr/en/museum-carnavalet/hotel-carnavalet/.

41 *"relié en peau humaine"*: *Constitution de la République Française…* (Dijon: Causse, 1793). Musée Carnavalet.

41 *Pierre-Charles de Villeneuve*: Etienne Taillemite, "Villeneuve, Pierre-Charles de (1763–1806), Vice Admiral," *Dictionnaire Napoléon* (Paris: Fayard, 1999), accessed November 9, 2017, https://www.napoleon.org/histoire-des-2-empires /biographies/villeneuve-pierre-charles-de-1763-1806-vice-amiral/.

41 *diplomat Louis Félix Étienne*: Sénat, "Turgot Louis-Félix-Étienne," March 8, 2016, accessed November 4, 2017, https://www.senat.fr/senateur-2nd-empire /turgot_louis_felix_etienne0252e2.html.

42 *its collections swell*: Kristian Jensen, *Revolution and the Antiquarian Book: Reshaping the Past, 1780–1815* (New York: Cambridge University Press, 2014), 12–13.

42 *viewed as fashionable objects*: David McKittrick, *The Invention of Rare Books: Private Interest and Public Memory, 1600–1840* (Cambridge, U.K.: Cambridge University Press, 2018), 232–33.

42 *began amassing as many incunabula*: Jensen, *Revolution and the Antiquarian Book*, 5.

42 *a surgeon named Cantin*: M. Doucin, *Histoire des vingt premières années de la Société Académique de Nantes et de la Loire-Inférieure* (Nantes: C. Mellinet, 1875), 27, https://books.google.com/books?id=HmA3AQAAMAAJ.

42 *"In denouncing the past"*: "En dénonçant le passé, nous voulons l'oublier; nous désirons réformer le présent et assurer un meilleur ordre pour l'avenir. Nous voulons, en un mot, que l'on ne confie plus le droit terrible de vie et de mort qu'à celui qui aura mérité la confiance publique en se livrant aux deux parties à la fois." Translation by the author. M. Cantin, *Projet de réforme adressé à l'Assemblée Nationale* (Paris: De l'impr. De Vezard, 1790), 6, https://hdl.handle.net/2027/ucm .5327673641.

43 *"I will admit"*: "J'admettrai néanmoins que nos anciens corps politiques étoient contraire à la liberté; mais ce vice tenoit à leur puissance et à leur organisation." Translation by the author. Cantin, *Projet de réforme*, 13–14.

43 *"If, under the pretext"*: "Si, sous prétexte d'une liberté indéfinie, on permettoit à tous ceux qui se croiroient médecins d'en faire les fonctions, ce seroit autoriser tous les impudens et tous lè les ignorans à n'être plus que des assassins impunis … il vaudroit bien mieux dès ce moment interdire l'exercice de la médecine.

On éviteroit du moins ces massacres journaliers, qui croîtroient en raison du dépérissement de l'art, et de là considération de ceux qui l'exercent." Translation by the author. Cantin, *Projet de réforme*, 15–16.

44 *years for some of Cantin's recommendations to be instituted*: Michel Foucault, *The Birth of the Clinic: An Archaeology of Medical Perception* (New York: Pantheon Books, 1973), 65.

44 *"The presence of disease"*: Foucault, *Birth of the Clinic*, xi.

45 *"But to look"*: Foucault, *Birth of the Clinic*, 84.

46 *the leather binding was horse*: *L'office de l'église en François* (Paris: Chez Pierre Le Petit, 1671). UC Berkeley Library, http://oskicat.berkeley.edu/record=b10357222~S6.

3. GENTLEMEN COLLECTORS

49 *twenty-eight-year-old Irish widow*: Beth Lander, "The Skin She Lived In: Anthropodermic Books in the Historical Medical Library," *Fugitive Leaves*, October 1, 2015, http://histmed.collegeofphysicians.org/skin-she-lived-in/.

49 *"being undermined by workmen"*: "Fearful Disaster in Philadelphia," *The New York Times*, July 21, 1864, accessed August 24, 2018, https://timesmachine.nytimes .com/timesmachine/1864/07/21/78727646.pdf.

50 *the young doctor*: John Stockton Hough, "Two Cases of Trichiniasis Observed at the Philadelphia Hospital, Blockley," *The American Journal of the Medical Sciences (1827–1924)* 114 (1869): 565.

50 *"Counting the number"*: Hough, "Two Cases," 565.

50 *in a chamber pot*: Lander, "Skin She Lived In."

50 *developed a speculum*: John Stockton Hough, "Description of a New Self-sustaining Vaginal, Uterine, and Anal Speculum Combined, for Examinations and Operations," *The American Journal of the Medical Sciences (1827–1924)* 116 (1869): 409.

51 *Dr. John Stockton Hough, like many gentlemen doctors*: Fred B. Rogers and Thomas A. Horrocks, "Dr. John Stockton Hough: Medical Bibliophile and Bibliographer," *Transactions of the College of Physicians of Philadelphia* 11 (1989): 355–56.

51 *He traveled to Europe*: Genevieve Miller. "'The Fielding H. Garrison Lecture': In Praise of Amateurs: Medical History in America Before Garrison," *Bulletin of the History of Medicine* 47, no. 6 (1973): 589.

51 *"foster the study"*: Grolier Club, "A Brief History of the Grolier Club," accessed November 19, 2019, https://www.grolierclub.org/Default.aspx?p =dynamicmodule&pageid=384895&ssid=322516&vnf=1.

51 *delighted in showing off*: Rogers, "Dr. John Stockton Hough," 358.

51 *he estimated in 1880*: "Biographical Sketch of John Stockton Hough," Historical Medical Library of the College of Physicians of Philadelphia.

51 *His copy of Fabricius*: Rogers, "Dr. John Stockton Hough," 359–60.

52 *Hough died at age fifty-six*: Rogers, "Dr. John Stockton Hough," 358.

52 *"This book is the biggest"*: John Pollack, interview with the author, September 29, 2015.

53 *that same Grolier Club*: Grolier Club, *Le traicté de Peyne* . . . (Paris: Librarie Rouquette, 1867), Grolier Club, http://grolier.vtls.com:3272/lib/item?id=chamo:19 318&theme=grolier/.

53 *red rot, an irreversible condition*: American Institute for Conservation of Art and Historic Works, "Red Rot," updated August 20, 2014, http://www.conservation -wiki.com/wiki/Red_rot/.

54 *"I feel like he picked"*: John Pollack, interview with the author, September 29, 2015.

54 *"The Bibliotheque National [sic]"*: Bibliothèque Impériale, *Catalog des sciences médicales* (Paris: Librarie de Firmin Didot Frères, Fils, Etc., 1861). Penn Libraries.

55 *"skin from around the wrist"*: Charles Drelincourt, *De conceptione adversaria* (London: Cornelium Boutestein, 1686). Historical Medical Library of the College of Physicians of Philadelphia.

55 *"T McC"*: Hough, "Two Cases," 565.

56 *Philadelphia General Hospital's Male Register*: Philadelphia General Hospital, Register of Males 1862–1868. Philadelphia City Archives.

56 *Leidy's Philadelphia*: Leonard Warren, *Joseph Leidy: The Last Man Who Knew Everything* (New Haven: Yale University Press, 1998), 18–19.

57 *poking at his breakfast ham*: Henry Fairfield Osborn, *Biographical Memoir of Joseph Leidy 1823–1891* (Washington, D.C.: National Academy of Sciences, 1913), 343.

57 *In the 1840s, the microscope*: Warren, *Joseph Leidy*, 28–29.

57 *a shy boy*: Joseph Leidy Jr., unpublished memoir, Historical Medical Library of the College of Physicians of Philadelphia, 8.

57 *But while Leidy's passion*: Warren, *Joseph Leidy*, 24–25.

57 *At the time that Leidy began*: Warren, *Joseph Leidy*, 125.

57 *"The profession"*: Warren, *Joseph Leidy*, 117.

58 *"For the general practitioner"*: William Osler, "Books and Men," in *Aequanimitas, with Other Addresses to Medical Students, Nurses, and Practitioners of Medicine*, 2nd ed. (Philadelphia: P. Blakiston's Son & Co., 1925), 221, http://www .medicalarchives.jhmi.edu/osler/booksandmen.htm.

58 *"We need more"*: Osler, "Books and Men," 223.

59 *"devoid of personal ambition"*: Osborn, *Biographical Memoir*, 348–49.

59 *"gentle, sympathethic"*: Leidy Jr., unpublished memoir, 19.

59 *"Quite simply"*: Warren, *Joseph Leidy*, xi–xii.

59 *"was so disgusted"*: Leidy Jr., unpublished memoir, 9.

59 *Legend has it*: Warren, *Joseph Leidy*, 46.

60 *He distinguished himself as a leader*: Osborn, *Biographical Memoir*, 361.

60 *earliest crimes solved by forensic means*: Warren, *Joseph Leidy*, 72.

60 *Back in the 1850s*: Warren, *Joseph Leidy*, 112.

60 *treated Nash*: Warren, *Joseph Leidy*, 113.

61 *Leidy advocated strongly*: Warren, *Joseph Leidy*, 118–19.

61 *Because he wanted*: Warren, *Joseph Leidy*, 129.

61 *Business at the medical school*: Warren, *Joseph Leidy*, 136.

61 *"If I had"*: Leidy Jr., unpublished memoir, 5–6.

61 *Satterlee military hospital*: Osborn, *Biographical Memoir*, 350.

62 *"human skin, from a soldier"*: Joseph Leidy, *An Elementary Treatise on Human Anatomy* (Philadelphia: J. B. Lippincott & Co., 1861), Historical Medical Library of the College of Physicians of Philadelphia.

62 *When his nephew's wife*: Helen Carter Leidy, letter to Dr. Packard, January 2, 1933, Historical Medical Library of the College of Physicians of Philadelphia.

62 *part of a worldwide network*: Warren, *Joseph Leidy*, 82.

63 *airless subterranean environment*: Anna N. Dhody, "The Curious Case of Mrs. Ellenbogen: Saponification and Deceit in 19th-Century Philadelphia," *Expedition Magazine* 58, no. 2 (2016), 45, http://www.penn.museum/sites/expedition /?p=23873/.

63 *"put on airs"*: Dhody, "Case of Mrs. Ellenbogen," 46–48.

63 *Leidy invoiced the museum*: Ella N. Wade, "A Curator's Story of the Mütter Museum and College Collections," *Transactions of the College of Physicians of Philadelphia* 42 (1974): 147.

63 *Leidy told the Mütter*: "No Lye: Docs Probe 'Soap Lady,'" *Wired*, September 28, 2001, https://www.wired.com/2001/09/no-lye-docs-probe-soap-lady/.

64 *"felt like we had"*: Allison Meier, "The Race to Rescue the Remains of an 18th-Century Cemetery," *Hyperallergic*, April 20, 2017, https://hyperallergic.com /373393/the-arch-street-bones-project/.

4. SKIN CRAFT

67 *few bookbinders*: Paul Kersten, "Bucheinbände in Menschenleder," in *Die Heftlade: Zeitschrift für die Förderer des Jakob Krausse-Bundes*, ed. Ernst Collin (Berlin: Euphorion Verlag, 1922–1924), 53–54.

68 *rarely written down*: Annick Vuissoz et al., "The Survival of PCR-Amplifiable DNA in Cow Leather," *Journal of Archaeological Science* 34 (2007): 825.

68 *almost no one*: Jesse Meyer, interview with the author, July 20, 2018.

68 *named after the ancient Greek city*: N. Poulakakis et al., "Ancient DNA and the Genetic Signature of Ancient Greek Manuscripts," *Journal of Archaeological Science* 34 (2007): 675.

69 *A food writer friend*: A few days after my visit to the tannery that food writer friend, Jonathan Gold, died. I am forever sad I'll never get to tell him that story. I highly recommend reading his Pulitzer Prize–winning work.

70 *once called Richard E. Meyer & Sons*: Pergamena, "About Us," accessed November 20, 2019, https://www.pergamena.net/about-us/.

70 *the business focused*: Jesse Meyer, interview with the author, July 20, 2018.

70 *environmental regulations*: Jesse Meyer, interview with the author, July 20, 2018.

71 *"You have a parchment"*: Jesse Meyer, interview with the author, July 20, 2018.

71 *"Although the use"*: Fiddyment et al., "Animal Origin of 13th-Century Uterine Vellum": 15070.

72 *"tanned in a 'pot de chambre'"*: Robert Couper, *Speculations on the Mode and Appearances of Impregnation in the Human Female* (Edinburgh: C. Elliot, 1789). Historical Medical Library of the College of Physicians of Philadelphia.

72 *may have added salt*: Jesse Meyer, interview with the author, July 20, 2018.

72 *added lime*: Jesse Meyer, interview with the author, July 20, 2018.

72 *lant*: "lant, n.1," in *OED Online* (Oxford University Press, 2019), accessed November 3, 2019, https://www.oed.com/view/Entry/105653.

72 *could take up to a week*: Jesse Meyer, interview with the author, July 20, 2018.

72 *human follicles are deeper*: Carolyn Marvin, "The Body of the Text: Literary's Corporeal Constant," *The Quarterly Journal of Speech* 80, no. 2 (1994): 134.

73 *used a draw knife*: Jesse Meyer, interview with the author, July 20, 2018.

73   *bating*: Jesse Meyer, interview with the author, July 20, 2018.

73   *tanned in sumac*: I. Sever. Pinaei, *De integritatis & corruptionis virginum notis* (Amsterdam: J. Ravestein: 1663). Wellcome Library, http://catalogue.wellcomelibrary .org/record=b1283248~S12.

73   *"It's a very nice smell"*: Jesse Meyer, interview with the author, July 20, 2018.

74   *librarian Beth Lander suggested*: Lander, "Skin She Lived In."

74   *contemporary Native Alaskan artists*: Smithsonian's National Museum of Natural History, "Material Traditions—Sewing Salmon," YouTube video, 6:21, July 17, 2013, https://www.youtube.com/watch?v=u38rPWITkjc.

74   *"Fish oils"*: Jesse Meyer, e-mail to the author, August 25, 2018.

74   *"I don't think"*: Jesse Meyer, e-mail to the author, August 26, 2018.

76   *"that feels like a big"*: Jesse Meyer, interview with the author, July 20, 2018.

5. SECRETS OF THE SAGES-FEMMES

79   *"Hush, hush, midwife"*: Bridgette Sheridan, "Childbirth, Midwifery, and Science: The Life and Work of the French Royal Midwife Louise Bourgeois (1563–1636)," Ph.D. diss., Boston College, 2002, 119–20.

79   *"Above all"*: P. M. Dunn, "Louise Bourgeois (1563–1636): Royal Midwife of France," *Archives of Disease in Childhood, Fetal & Neonatal Edition* 85 (2004): F186.

80   *The wife of an assistant to the legendary surgeon Ambroise Paré*: Jennifer S. Uglow et al., eds., "Bourgeois, Louyse," in *The Palgrave Macmillan Dictionary of Women's Biography*, 4th ed. (New York: Palgrave Macmillan, 2005).

80   *"If [the midwife]"*: Dunn, "Louise Bourgeois," F186.

80   *The top of the title page*: Louise Bourgeois, *Observations diverses sur la stérilité, perte de fruict, foecondité...* (Paris: Chez A. Saugrain, 1609), http://gallica.bnf.fr /ark:/12148/btv1b8401326n/.

80   *The 1621 edition*: Jacques Guillemeau and Charles Guillemeau, *De la grossesse et accouchement des femmes . . .* (Paris: A. Pacard, 1621), http://gallica.bnf.fr/ark: /12148/bpt6k5701564n/.

81   *"recognize in it*: "Les sages femmes pourront aussi jouir de pareil benefice, & sans s'amuser à la vanité de leur art, y recognoistre à bon escient plusieurs defauts en ce qui concerne la dexterité des accouchemens, & la guarison des accouchées." Translation by the author. Guillemeau and Guillemeau, *De la grossesse* (unnumbered page).

81   *As the historian Bridgette Sheridan asserts*: Sheridan, "Childbirth," 70.

81   *After the assassination of King Henry IV*: Paul Lagasse, "Louis XIII, king of France," in *The Columbia Encyclopedia*, 8th ed. (New York: Columbia University Press, 2018).

82   *Marie de Médicis ordered an autopsy*: Louise Bourgeois, "Fidelle relation de l'accouchement, maladie & ouverture du corps de feu madame," (1627), https:// gallica.bnf.fr/ark:/12148/bpt6k5440853z/. Note: This online edition with a different title is identical to another version published in 1627 called "Apologie de Louyse Bourgeois dite Bourcier sage femme de la Royne Mere du Roy, et de feu Madame. Contre le Rapport des Medicins." This document is commonly referred to as the Apologie.

82   *In those days, autopsy reports*: Louise Bourgeois Boursier, *Recit veritable de la naissance de messeigneurs et dames les enfans de France*, ed. François Rouget and

Colette H. Winn (Paris: Librarie Droz, 2000), 104n24, https://books.google
.com/books?id=4qRWDdYNe8YC.

82 *likely acute peritonitis*: Boursier, *Recit veritable*, 104n22.

82 *"Based on your report"*: "Par vostre rapport vous faictes affez cognoistre, que vous
n'entendez rien du tout en la cognoiffance de l'arrierefaix et de la matrice d'vne
femme, tant auant, qu'apres fon accouchement; non plus que vostre Maistre
Galien, lequel pour n'auoir jamais esté marié, et auoir peu affisté en leur accouchement, s'estant meflé d'enseigner vne fage-femme par vn liure, qu'il a faict
exprés, il a faict parestre, qu'il n'a iamais cognu la matrice d'vne femme enceinte,
ny mefmes fon arriere-faix." Translation by the author. Bourgeois, "Fidelle relation," 7.

83 *"to know the secrets"*: "Mais pour fçavoir les fecrets des maladies des femmes, il
faut auoir frequenté les fages-femmes, et auoir assisté à plufieurs accouchemens,
comme auoit fait vostre grand Maistre et legiflateur Hippocrate, qui au fait des
maladies des femmes, confultoit les fages-femmes, s'en rapportoit à leur iuge-
ment." Translation by the author. Bourgeois, "Fidelle relation," 17.

83 *historians attribute the writing to Charles Guillemeau*: Sheridan, "Childbirth,"
143n 47.

83 *"You should rather"*: "You should rather have spent the rest of your life without
speaking, than to claim as you do . . . that this great Princess was not as well
taken care of as she should have been . . . Consider these things, M. [Bourgeois]
Bourcier [*sic*] and contain yourself within the limits of your duty—no longer
involve yourself in correcting Physicians." Translation by Sheridan, "Childbirth," 143–44.

83 *"preservatif infaillible"*: Louise Bourgeois Boursier, *Recueil des secrets de Louyse
Bourgeois, dite Boursier*... (Paris: M. Mondière: 1635), 4–6, accessed October 10,
2018, via Proquest Early European Books database.

84 *dubbed* vielles: Alison Klairmont Lingo, "Empirics and Charlatans in Early
Modern France: The Genesis of the Classification of the 'Other' in Medical Practice," *Journal of Social History* 19 (1986): 596.

84 *André du Breil*: Lingo, "Empirics," 591.

84 *Women medical practitioners are perceived*: Christina Klöckner Cronauer and
Marianne Schmid Mast, "Hostile Sexist Male Patients and Female Doctors: A
Challenging Encounter," *Patient* 7 (2014): 38.

85 *Of the nearly six thousand women doctors surveyed*: Elizabeth Fernandez, "Physician Moms Are Often Subject to Workplace Discrimination," *UCSF News Center*, May 8, 2017, accessed October 19, 2018, https://www.ucsf.edu/news/2017/05
/406921/physician-moms-are-often-subject-workplace-discrimination/.

85 *The tasteful Persian*: Development Communications, "Scheide Donates Rare
Books Library to Princeton; Collection Is Largest Gift in University's History,"
Princeton University, February 16, 2015, accessed December 11, 2017, https://www
.princeton.edu/news/2015/02/16/scheide-donates-rare-books-library-princeton
-collection-largest-gift-universitys.

85 *The glass bookcases*: Department of Rare Books and Special Collections, "Scheide
Library," *Princeton University Library*, accessed December 11, 2017, https://rbsc
.princeton.edu/divisions/scheide-library.

86 *"I don't like"*: Paul Needham, interview with the author, September 28, 2015.

86 *"Of course he chose"*: Paul Needham, interview with the author, September 28, 2015.

87 *"I am pretty permanently"*: Paul Needham, interview with the author, September 28, 2015.

87 *European rag paper suppliers*: Nicholson Baker, *Double Fold: Libraries and the Assault on Paper* (New York: Vintage Books, 2001), 61–64.

88 *"I agree that librarians"*: Paul Needham, interview with the author, September 28, 2015.

90 *Shortly after my visit*: Rosaline Crone, "Jack the Ripper, a Women's History Museum and London's Fascination with All Things Gory," *The Conversation*, July 31, 2015, https://theconversation.com/jack-the-ripper-a-womens-history-museum -and-londons-fascination-with-all-things-gory-45456/.

91 *one of the Dungeon's skeletons*: "London Dungeon Skeleton Found to Be Real," *BBC News*, December 5, 2011, http://www.bbc.com/news/uk-england-london -1603750/.

92 *"They're historical artifacts"*: Elma Brenner, interview with the author, July 22, 2015.

6. THE LONG SHADOW OF THE NIGHT DOCTORS

95 *Attucks was born into enslavement*: Crispus Attucks Museum, "Biography of Crispus Attucks," September 12, 2012, accessed October 6, 2018, http://www .crispusattucksmuseum.org/biography/.

95 *Crispus Attucks and the four other men*: Crispus Attucks Museum, "Where is Crispus Attucks buried?," February 17, 2013, accessed October 6, 2018, http://www .crispusattucksmuseum.org/where-is-crispus-attucks-buried/.

96 *"The cover of this book"*: Wellcome Collection, "A Notebook Allegedly Covered in Human Skin . . . ," accessed November 1, 2018, https://wellcomecollection .org/works/yj2tzxt6/.

96 *Wellcome earned an incalculable fortune*: Science Museum, "Henry Wellcome (1853–1936)," *Brought to Life: Exploring the History of Medicine*, accessed October 6, 2018, http://broughttolife.sciencemuseum.org.uk/broughttolife/people /henrywellcome/.

96 *coined the word* tabloid: Frances Larson, "The Things About Henry Wellcome," *Journal of Material Culture* 15, no. 1 (March 22, 2010): 86–87.

96 *the largest private museum collection in the world*: Larson, "Things About Henry," 83.

96 *vigilant regarding fakes*: Larson, "Things About Henry," 98.

97 *purchased the book for £3*: Wellcome Library acquisitions book, 1930–1947, accessed October 19, 2018, https://wellcomelibrary.org/item/b28477637#?c=0&m=0&s =0&cv=284&z=-0.4139%2C-0.0625%2C1.6335%2C1.1101.

97 *roughly $170 today*: Using a currency converter (http://www.nationalarchives .gov.uk/currency-converter/#currency-result) set to 1930, 3 pounds is equivalent in 2017 purchasing power to £137.36. Then I used the IRS yearly average exchange rate for the U.K. in 2017 (0.808) and followed their instructions to divide the foreign currency amount by the applicable yearly average exchange rate to convert from foreign currency to U.S. dollars, resulting in $170. See https://www.irs.gov /individuals/international-taxpayers/yearly-average-currency-exchange-rates. The most recent year available using this tool is 2017.

97 *"The hair follicle"*: Christopher Calnan (The National Trust for Places of Historic Interest or Natural Beauty) letter to Tony Bish (Wellcome Trust), August 12, 2002, copy provided by Wellcome Library. The "(?)" included in the quote is original to the letter.

98 *Art forgers are often motivated*: Noah Charney, *The Art of Forgery: The Minds, Motives and Methods of Master Forgers* (New York: Phaidon Press, 2015), 14.

98 *human skin book frauds*: Charney, *Art of Forgery*, 17–18.

98 *leaving fake information*: Charney, *Art of Forgery*, 177.

99 *Giovanni Pico della Mirandola*: M. V. Dougherty, "Giovanni Pico Della Mirandola," in *Encyclopedia of Medieval Philosophy: Philosophy Between 500 and 1500*, ed. Henrik Lagerlund (Dordrecht: Springer, 2011).

100 *"So this fella"*: Liz Dube and George Rugg, interview with the author, October 12, 2015.

100 *Bookworms*: Andrijana Sajic, "A Book's Best Frenemy," *In Circulation*, February 24, 2016, https://www.metmuseum.org/blogs/in-circulation/2016/book-lovers/.

101 *"Some sort of rodent"*: Liz Dube and George Rugg, interview with the author, October 12, 2015.

101 *"This old Tome"*: Giovanni Pico della Mirandola, *Opera Joannis Pici Mirandule . . .* (Argentinus: Ioannes Prüs Ciuis Argentinus, 1503), University of Notre Dame Hesburgh Libraries, https://onesearch.library.nd.edu/permalink/f/tgve9/ndu_aleph000943748.

101 *"Do not get frightened"*: John Nagy, "The Truth Uncovered," *Notre Dame Magazine*, accessed August 28, 2018, https://magazine.nd.edu/news/65313/.

102 *Coralla was the intended target*: "Religion Costs Lives Texan Kills Wife and Self as Result of Quarrel," *Oregonian*, March 8, 1916, 2.

102 *"People went about"*: "Quake Fails to Materialize," *Dallas Morning News*, April 21, 1908, 12.

102 *"It could conceivably"*: Liz Dube and George Rugg, interview with the author, October 12, 2015.

103 *my team tested the book*: Nagy, "The Truth Uncovered."

103 *"The title leather"*: Dale Carnegie, *Lincoln the Unknown* (New York and London: The Century Co., 1932). Temple University Libraries.

104 *"The compositions published"*: Henry Louis Gates Jr., *The Trials of Phillis Wheatley: America's First Black Poet and Her Encounters with the Founding Fathers* (New York: Basic Civitas, 2003), 42–43.

105 *"Essentially"*: Gates, *Trials of Phillis*, 27.

105 *no American publisher*: Gates, *Trials of Phillis*, 31.

105 *She was gifted*: Harvard Library, "Paradise Lost, a Poem," accessed November 2, 2018, http://id.lib.harvard.edu/alma/990029682250203941/catalog/.

105 *"a person so favored"*: Gates, *Trials of Phillis*, 38.

105 *When Phillis Wheatley's book*: Gates, *Trials of Phillis*, 34.

105 *She placed ads in Boston*: Gates, *Trials of Phillis*, 66–68.

106 *her husband sold*: Harvard Library, *Paradise Lost*.

106 *the Wheatley human skin books*: "Preservation Lab-Examination and Treatment Report," *The Preservation Lab: A Collaboration of the Public Library of Cincinnati & Hamilton County and the University of Cincinnati Libraries*, November 3, 2015, accessed August 29, 2018, https://drc.libraries.uc.edu

/bitstream/handle/2374.UC/749881/i29412262_1052_PLCH_TrtRpt_Wheatley
.pdf?sequence=7/.

106 *whose Metuchen*: Gary A. Donaldson, "The Career of Charles F. Heartman and the Tradition of Collecting Americana," *The Papers of the Bibliographical Society of America* 84, no. 4 (1990): 384, http://www.jstor.org/stable/24303060/.

107 *"a little fuehrer"*: Donaldson, "Career of Charles F. Heartman": 382.

107 *a four-hundred-acre plot*: Donaldson, "Career of Charles F. Heartman": 389.

107 *the Book Farm did not work out*: Peggy Price, "The Book Farm: Charles F. Heartman's Utopia for Intellectuals," *Fine Books Magazine*, April 2010, accessed September 2, 2018, https://www.finebooksmagazine.com/issue/201004/heartman-1.phtml, 2.

107 *Heartman found the book collections*: Donaldson, "Career of Charles F. Heartman," 388–90.

107 *He also created and sold reprints*: Donaldson, "Career of Charles F. Heartman," 393.

107 *created a bibliography*: Arthur A. Schomburg, *A Bibliographical Checklist of American Negro Poetry* (New York: C. F. Heartman, 1916).

107 *"a man with a big heart"*: Arthur A. Schomburg, "A Bibliophile," *The Crisis* 11 no. 1 (November 1915): 14, https://www.marxists.org/history/usa/workers/civil-rights/crisis/1100-crisis-v11n01-w061.pdf.

108 *Wheatleys "using leather supplied"*: Zaehnsdorf invoice, M94 Charles F. Heartman Papers, M94, Box 5, Folder 7, Historical Manuscripts, Special Collections, the University of Southern Mississippi Libraries.

108 *"For me"*: Michael Joseph, Rutgers University, personal correspondence with Richard Hark, November 15, 2015. Quoted with permission from Michael Joseph.

108 *just under $300*: I calculated this figure by using the National Archives Currency Converter: 1270–2017, www.nationalarchives.gov.uk/currency-converter/, for the year 1935 (closest date available) to equal £234.95 in 2017. Then I used the IRS yearly average exchange rate for the U.K. in 2017 (0.808) and followed their instructions to divide the foreign currency amount by the applicable yearly average exchange rate to convert from foreign currency to U.S. dollars, resulting in $290.78. See https://www.irs.gov/individuals/international-taxpayers/yearly-average-currency-exchange-rates.

109 *"The literary work"*: Charles F. Heartman, *Phillis Wheatley (Phillis Peters); A Critical Attempt and a Bibliography of Her Writings* (New York, 1915), 27, https://archive.org/details/philliswheatleypoohear/.

110 *a trophy-taking practice*: Simon Harrison, "Skull Trophies of the Pacific War: Transgressive Objects of Remembrance," *Journal of the Royal Anthropological Institute* 12, no. 4 (2006): 818–20.

110 *the Night Doctors*: Harriet A. Washington, *Medical Apartheid: The Dark History of Medical Experimentation on Black Americans from Colonial Times to the Present* (New York: Anchor Books, 2006), 119.

110 *Doctors openly placed ads*: Daina Ramey Berry, *The Price for Their Pound of Flesh: The Value of the Enslaved, from Womb to Grave, in the Building of a Nation* (Boston: Beacon Press, 2017), 167.

111 *"medical nonentity"*: Washington, *Medical Apartheid*, 46.

111 *lynching mementos often included photos*: Washington, *Medical Apartheid*, 136.

111 *photos of medical school students*: For an excellent work about this practice, see John Harley Warner and James M. Edmonson, *Dissection: Photographs of a Rite of Passage in American Medicine, 1880–1930* (New York: Blast Books, 2009).

111 *"Fortunately, the facts"*: Washington, *Medical Apartheid*, 10.

111 *The Tuskegee Syphilis Study*: Centers for Disease Control and Prevention, "The Tuskegee Timeline," updated December 22, 2015, https://www.cdc.gov/tuskegee /timeline.htm/.

111 *The Black body*: Washington, *Medical Apartheid*, 138–39.

111 *Doctors' biases toward Black patients*: Kelly M. Hoffman et al., "Racial Bias in Pain Assessment and Treatment Recommendations, and False Beliefs About Biological Differences Between Blacks and Whites," *PNAS* 113, no. 16 (2016): 4296.

112 *"There's a long history"*: Jillian Tullis, e-mail to the author, October 27, 2018.

112 *Albert Monroe Wilson*: Penn University Archives and Records Center, "Albert Monroe Wilson 1841–1904," accessed February 11, 2020, https://archives.upenn .edu/exhibits/penn-people/biography/albert-monroe-wilson.

113 *quietly aiding the cadaver trade*: Berry, *Pound of Flesh*, 190–91.

7. THE POSTMORTEM TRAVELS OF WILLIAM CORDER

115 *her neighbor's Red Barn*: Ron Murrell, interview with the author, July 15, 2015.

115 *had recently borne another by Corder*: The *Trial of William Corder, at the Assizes, Bury St. Edmunds, Suffolk, August 7th and 8th, 1828, for The Murder of Maria Marten, in The Red Barn, at Polstead* ... (London: Knight & Lacey, 1828), 29.

115 *Corder told the Martens*: *Trial of William Corder*, 34–35.

115 *"If I go to gaol"*: *Trial of William Corder*, 29.

116 *he saw Corder leave the barn alone*: *Trial of William Corder*, 34–35.

116 *"No, she is not," Corder replied*: *Trial of William Corder*, 30–31.

117 *Unusually for the daughter*: Ron Murrell, interview with the author, July 15, 2015.

117 *Corder explained that she was afflicted*: *Trial of William Corder*, 34–35.

117 *"I think, were I in your place"*: J. Curtis, *The Murder of Maria Marten: Being an Authentic and Faithful History with a Full Development of the Most Extraordinary Circumstances Which Led to the Discovery of Her Body in the Red Barn* ... (New York: Pellegrini & Cudahy, 1948), 54.

117 *Thomas Marten grabbed his mole spud*: Ron Murrell, interview with the author, July 15, 2015.

117 *green kerchief still tied*: Curtis, *Murder of Maria Marten*, 69–70.

117 *Her combs and earrings*: *Trial of William Corder*, 11–12.

117 *A local surgeon made notes*: Curtis, *Murder of Maria Marten*, 113.

117 *her rotting hand dropped*: *Trial of William Corder*, 19.

118 *"chief of his family"*: *Trial of William Corder*, 7–9.

118 *The officer asked Corder three times*: *Trial of William Corder*, 33.

118 *Reporters flocked*: Curtis, *Murder of Maria Marten*, 65.

118 *Near the Red Barn, a preacher*: Curtis, *Murder of Maria Marten*, 130.

118 *nearly five thousand onlookers*: *Trial of William Corder*, 59.

118 *William Corder's mother*: Curtis, *Murder of Maria Marten*, 79–80.

118 *Rain poured down*: *Trial of William Corder*, 45.

119 *"He's coming!"*: Curtis, *Murder of Maria Marten*, 99–101.

119 *court proceedings had to pause*: Curtis, *Murder of Maria Marten*, 136.

119 *When court adjourned*: Curtis, *Murder of Maria Marten*, 143–45.

119 *one upper-class woman told a reporter*: Curtis, *Murder of Maria Marten*, 208.

119 *After denouncing his unfair treatment*: *Trial of William Corder*, 49.

119 *Prosecutors called his explanation ludicrous*: *Trial of William Corder*, 55.

119 *Corder dropped his chin*: Curtis, *Murder of Maria Marten*, 175.

119 *"William Corder"*: Curtis, *Murder of Maria Marten*, 175–77.

120 *The habitual hanging tree*: Curtis, *Murder of Maria Marten*, 186.

120 *Hanging offenses varied greatly*: Ruth Richardson, *Death, Dissection, and the Destitute* (Chicago: University of Chicago Press, 2000), 52–53.

121 *Corder wrote his confession*: Curtis, *Murder of Maria Marten*, 197.

121 *some ten thousand pairs of eyes*: Ron Murrell, interview with the author, July 15, 2015.

121 *Corder scarcely had time*: Curtis, *Murder of Maria Marten*, 207.

121 *"What I got"*: Curtis, *Murder of Maria Marten*, 210.

121 *An hour after William*: Curtis, *Murder of Maria Marten*, 211.

122 *Dr. Creed made it*: Ron Murrell, interview with the author, July 15, 2015.

122 *"Thus I shall be"*: Curtis, *Murder of Maria Marten*, 212.

122 *"I had a great pleasure"*: Curtis, *Murder of Maria Marten*, 214–15.

123 *Relic hunters stripped*: Ron Murrell, interview with the author, July 15, 2015.

123 *the murderer shifts*: Jack Denham, "The Commodification of the Criminal Corpse: 'Selective Memory' in Posthumous Representations of Criminal," *Mortality* 21, no. 3 (2016): 240.

124 *At Bristol's M Shed museum*: Fay Curtis, "The John Horwood Book," *Bristol's Free Museums and Historic Houses*, April 17, 2014, https://www.bristolmuseums.org.uk/blog/archives/john-horwood-book/.

124 *In Devon*: Jemima Laing, "Book Bound in Human Skin Goes on Display in Devon," *BBC Devon*, February 25, 2011, accessed March 30, 2018, http://www.bbc.com/news/uk-england-devon-12539388/.

124 *scratches a psychological itch*: Denham, "Commodification of the Criminal Corpse," 229–30.

124 *twelfth-century building*: Moyse's Hall Museum, "About," accessed March 30, 2018, https://www.moyseshall.org/about/.

124 *A gibbet*: Maryrose Cuskelly, *Original Skin: Exploring the Marvels of the Human Hide* (Berkeley, CA: Counterpoint, 2011), 157.

125 *An Act of Parliament in 1752*: Richardson, *Death, Dissection, and the Destitute*, 35–36.

125 *mummified cats and the "witch bottles"*: Brian Hoggard, "The Archaeology of Counter-Witchcraft and Popular Magic," in *Beyond the Witchtrials: Witchcraft and Magic in Enlightenment Europe*, ed. Owen Davies and William De Blécourt (Manchester, U.K.: Manchester University Press: 2004), 167.

126 *"People still come"*: Ron Murrell, interview with the author, July 15, 2015.

126 *"They used to take the skeleton"*: Ron Murrell, interview with the author, July 15, 2015.

126 *For centuries, the human skull*: Stanley B. Burns and Elizabeth A. Burns, *Stiffs, Skulls & Skeletons: Medical Photography and Symbolism* (Arglen, PA: Schiffer Publishing, 2014), 25.

126 *"the Student's Dream"*: For an example, see Warner and Edmonson, *Dissection*, 144–45.

126 *sword fighting with severed limbs*: Lindsey Fitzharris, *The Butchering Art: Joseph Lister's Quest to Transform the Grisly World of Victorian Medicine* (New York: Farrar, Straus and Giroux, 2017), 40.

127 *Linda Nessworthy*: Linda Nessworthy wrote a book in 2001 called *Murdering Maria: The Life & Trial of William Corder the Red Barn Murderer* (Great Yarmouth: Malinda Publishing, 2001).

127 *Museum officials did not want*: Simon Chaplin, interview with the author, July 22, 2015.

127 *"It was almost"*: "Killer Cremated After 180 Years," *BBC News*, August 17, 2004, accessed March 30, 2018, http://news.bbc.co.uk/2/hi/uk_news/england/suffolk /3573244.stm/.

127 *Emboldened by her success*: Cuskelly, *Original Skin*, 172–73.

128 *"Museums should make"*: Simon Chaplin, interview with the author, July 22, 2015.

128 *"I'm very comfortable"*: Simon Chaplin, interview with the author, July 22, 2015.

8. ECHOES OF TANNER'S CLOSE

131 *twenty-five thousand Scots*: John Baxter, "Unmaking a Murderer," *The Anatomy Lab* (blog), Surgeons' Hall Museums, January 27, 2017, accessed April 4, 2018, https://surgeonshallmuseums.wordpress.com/2017/01/27/unmaking-a-murderer/.

131 *"Burke him!"*: Surgeons' Hall Museums, "Execution of William Burke," https:// museum.rcsed.ac.uk/the-collection/key-collections/key-object-page?objID= 1227&page=2/.

131 *Tanner's Close*: Lisa Rosner, *Anatomy Murders: Being the True and Spectacular History of Edinburgh's Notorious Burke and Hare and the Man of Science Who Abetted Them in Their Most Heinous Crimes* (Philadelphia: University of Pennsylvania Press, 2010), 22.

131 *The method could not be identified as murder*: Rosner, *Anatomy Murders*, 55–56.

132 *"Burking Mania"*: Druin Burch, *Digging Up the Dead: Uncovering the Life and Times of an Extraordinary Surgeon* (London: Vintage Books, 2008), 238.

132 *"the area of the classroom"*: *West Port Murders; or An Authentic Account of the Atrocious Murders Committed by Burke and His Associates . . .* (Edinburgh: Thomas Ireland, Jr., 1829), 253–54, https://archive.org/details/b20443304/.

132 *probably a student*: Tom Rowley, "Edinburgh University Student 'Wrote Note with Serial Killer William Burke's Blood'," *The Telegraph*, May 4, 2015, accessed October 29, 2018, https://www.telegraph.co.uk/news/uknews/crime/11581641 /Edinburgh-University-student-wrote-note-with-serial-killer-William-Burkes -blood.html.

132 *Royal College of Surgeons of Edinburgh's*: Surgeons' Hall Museums, "Pocketbook Made from Burke's Skin," accessed October 27, 2018, https://museum.rcsed.ac .uk/the-collection/key-collections/key-object-page/pocketbook-made-from -burkes-skin/.

132 *the Surgeons' Hall Museums were closed*: The Royal College of Surgeons of Edinburgh, "Surgeons' Hall Museums Reopen After Major Transformation," September 24, 2015, accessed October 27, 2018 https://www.rcsed.ac.uk/news -public-affairs/news/2015/september/surgeons-hall-museums-reopen-after-major -transformation/.

133 *first crack at any bodies*: Rosner, *Anatomy Murders*, 29.

133 *rest on his family name*: Rosner, *Anatomy Murders*, 30.

133 *hands-on dissection experience was required*: Rosner, *Anatomy Murders*, 150.

133 *A younger generation*: Rosner, *Anatomy Murders*, 31.

133 *an inveterate body snatcher*: MacGregor, *History of Burke and Hare and of the Resurrectionist Times*, (Glasgow: Thomas D. Morison, 1884), 28–29, https://archive .org/details/historyofburkeha1884macg.

134 *a man named Donald*: *West Port Murders*, 331.

134 *one hundred days' pay*: Rosner, *Anatomy Murders*, 69.

134 *Joseph the Miller*: *West Port Murders*, 333.

135 *more than four hundred students*: Rosner, *Anatomy Murders*, 150.

135 *Smallpox-induced blindness*: Andrew S. Currie, "Robert Knox, Anatomist, Scientist, and Martyr," *Proceedings of the Royal Society of Medicine* 26, no. 1 (1932): 39.

135 *frills, lace, and diamond rings*: Rosner, *Anatomy Murders*, 158.

135 *"When a 'subject' was in the room"*: Rosner, *Anatomy Murders*, 96.

135 *"It seemed incredible"*: Rosner, *Anatomy Murders*, 80.

136 *anatomized victims were subsequently destroyed*: Richardson, *Death, Dissection, and the Destitute*, 133.

136 *created an effigy of Dr. Knox*: Richardson, *Death, Dissection, and the Destitute*, 138.

136 *Many of Knox's neighbors*: Rosner, *Anatomy Murders*, 249.

136 *"The Echo of Surgeons Square"*: The Echo of Surgeons Square, "Letter to the Lord Advocate, Disclosing the Accomplices, Secrets, and Other Facts Relative to the Late Murders" (Edinburgh, 1829), https://archive.org/details/b20443900/.

137 *A physician-led Committee*: Rosner, *Anatomy Murders*, 254–56.

137 *the Select Committee on Anatomy*: House of Commons, "Report from the Select Committee on Anatomy" (London, 1828), https://archive.org/details /reportfromselectoogrea/.

137 *In 1826, London's twelve*: Richardson, *Death, Dissection, and the Destitute*, 54.

138 *One French Benthamite*: Richardson, *Death, Dissection, and the Destitute*, 168.

138 *Transcripts of the Select Committee's*: Richardson, *Death, Dissection, and the Destitute*, 107–108.

138 *"the bodies of persons found dead"*: House of Commons, "Report from the Select Committee," 124.

139 *"a monstrous act"*: Richardson, *Death, Dissection, and the Destitute*, 145.

139 *"I would recommend"*: Richardson, *Death, Dissection, and the Destitute*, 100.

139 *"The Midnight Bill"*: R. Gibson, "Anatomy Bill," *The Lancet* 12, no. 301 (June 6, 1829): 319.

140 *"These interferences"*: House of Commons, "Report from the Select Committee," 127.

140 *Dr. Knox continued*: Rosner, *Anatomy Murders*, 40–41.

140 *Then, in November 1831*: Richardson, *Death, Dissection, and the Destitute*, 193.

140 *Warburton rendered the tone*: Richardson, *Death, Dissection, and the Destitute*, 198.

141 *One major proposed change*: "The Anatomy Act, 1832; The Pharmacy Act, 1852; The Pharmacy Act, 1869; The Anatomy Act, 1871," 905, https://archive.org/details /b21520483/.

141 *If a doctor did not abide by the new Anatomy Act*: "Anatomy Act, 1832," 906.

141 *a punishment for grave robbing*: Richardson, *Death, Dissection, and the Destitute*, 208.

141 *not considered property*: "Anatomy Act, 1832," 904.

142 *"I had the . . . difficult task"*: Richardson, *Death, Dissection, and the Destitute*, xiv.

142 *"There cannot have been"*: Richardson, *Death, Dissection, and the Destitute*, 207.

143 *"the lowest dregs of degradation"*: House of Commons, "Report from the Select Committee," 18.

143 *In September 1832*: Katrina Navickas, *Protest and the Politics of Space and Place, 1789–1848* (Manchester, U.K.: Manchester University Press, 2017), 132–34.

143 *Two thousand people*: Richardson, *Death, Dissection, and the Destitute*, 228–29.

144 *"that the disclosures"*: Richardson, *Death, Dissection, and the Destitute*, 97–98.

144 *"The indications are that"*: Richardson, *Death, Dissection, and the Destitute*, 255.

144 *The twentieth century saw a slow increase*: Richardson, *Death, Dissection, and the Destitute*, 259–60.

9. THE HIGHWAYMAN'S GIFT

147 *a suit and twelve dollars*: George Walton, *Narrative of the Life of James Allen, Alias George Walton, Alias Jonas Pierce, Alias James H. York, Alias Burley Grove the Highwayman. Being His Death-bed Confession, to the Warden of the Massachusetts State Prison* (Boston: Harrington & Co., 1837), 19. Boston Athenæum, https://cdm.bostonathenaeum.org/digital/collection/p15482coll3/id/4273.

147 *Walton used the money*: Walton, *Narrative*, 19.

147–48 *He grew up desperately poor*: Stephen Z. Nonack, "Narrative of the Life of James Allen, Alias George Walton, Alias Jonas Pierce, Alias James H. York, Alias Burley Grove the Highwayman. Being His Death-bed Confession, to the Warden of the Massachusetts State Prison," in *Acquired Tastes: 200 Years of Collecting for the Boston Athenæum*, ed. Stanley Ellis Cushing and David B. Dearinger (Boston: Boston Athenæum, 2007), 152.

148 *helped a man carry a suspicious package*: Walton, *Narrative*, 153.

148 *"The idea of being in prison"*: Walton, *Narrative*, 5.

148 *"I never, in my life"*: Walton, *Narrative*, 9.

149 *after getting caught digging*: Walton, *Narrative*, 13.

149 *garner a pardon in 1830*: Walton, *Narrative*, 14.

149 *stabbed in the head*: Walton, *Narrative*, 27–28.

149 *"I did not go out of prison"*: Walton, *Narrative*, 19.

150 *"Your money or your life!"*: Walton, *Narrative*, 15.

150 *"I thought, on his attacking me"*: Walton, *Narrative*, 23.

151 *"In Hosp. several times"*: Charles Lincoln Jr., *Diary of Charles Lincoln Jr.* (Boston, 1826–1842). Boston Athenæum.

151 *he was liked by both*: Walton, *Narrative*, 5.

151 *He died decades before*: For a look at the long road to our modern understanding of consumption, phthisis, and tuberculosis, see Basel H. Herzog, "History of Tuberculosis," *Respiration* 65 (1998): 5–15.

151 *"was not aware of being suspected"*: Walton, *Narrative*, 23.

152 *"At this stage of the narrative"*: Walton, *Narrative*, 30.

152 *"the infidel sentiments"*: Walton, *Narrative*, 31.

152 *The warden claimed that Walton told him*: Walton, *Narrative*, 32.

153 *"of a religious and moral character"*: Nonack, *Walton*, 153–54.

153 *he asked to see John Fenno*: Nonack, *Walton*, 153.

153 *tanned to resemble gray deerskin*: Nonack, *Walton*, 154.

154 *"Hic liber Waltonis"*: Walton, *Narrative of the Life of James Allen.*

154 *according to family lore*: Stanley Cushing, interview with the author, April 14, 2015.

154 *Around 1864, Fenno's daughter*: Nonack, *Walton*, 154.

154 *one of the oldest independent libraries*: Boston Athenæum, "Mission & History," accessed November 23, 2019, http://www.bostonathenaeum.org/about/mission -history/.

155 *"ooze" binding*: Geoffrey Glaister, "Ooze Leather," in *Encyclopedia of the Book* (New Castle, DE: Oak Knoll Press, 1996), quoted in University of Alabama, "Glossary H–O," *Publishers' Bindings Online, 1815–1930: The Art of Books* (2005), http://bindings.lib.ua.edu/glossary2.html.

155 *"You don't really want"*: Stanley Cushing, interview with the author, April 14, 2015.

155 *"He was a very handsome"*: Stanley Cushing, interview with the author, April 14, 2015.

156 *found not guilty by reason of insanity*: George Tyler Bigelow and George Bemis, *Report of the Trial of Abner Rogers, Jr: Indicted for the Murder of Charles Lincoln, JR., Late Warden of the Massachusetts State Prison; Before the Supreme Judicial Court of Massachusetts, Holden at Boston, on Tuesday, January 30, 1844* (Boston: Charles C. Little and James Brown, 1844).

156 *threw himself out of a window*: Bigelow, *Trial of Abner Rogers*, 283.

157 *"a twenty-first-century"*: David Pearson, *Provenance Research in Book History: A Handbook* (New Castle, DE: Oak Knoll Press, 2019), 6–7.

157 *"I see no reason"*: Stanley Cushing, interview with the author, April 14, 2015.

158 *If a prisoner is executed or dies*: Manny Fernandez, "Texas Prisoner Burials Are a Gentle Touch in a Punitive System," *The New York Times*, January 4, 2012, www .nytimes.com/2012/01/05/us/texas-prisoner-burials-are-a-gentle-touch-in-a -punitive-system.html

158 *"I think everyone assumes"*: Fernandez, "Texas Prisoner."

159 *"The first law of nature"*: Walton, *Narrative*, 8.

10. GHOSTS IN THE LIBRARY

161 *On May 10, 1933*: United States Holocaust Memorial Museum, "Book Burning," Holocaust Encyclopedia, accessed July 27, 2018, https://www.ushmm.org/wlc /en/article.php?ModuleId=10005852/.

161 *the Deutsche Studentenschaft*: Anders Rydell, *The Book Thieves: The Nazi Looting of Europe's Libraries and the Race to Return a Literary Inheritance* (New York: Viking, 2017), 2.

161 *storm troopers, disguised in black tie*: Rydell, *Book Thieves*, 2.

161 *coined the term* Third Reich: Rydell, *Book Thieves*, 46.

162 *"No to decadence"*: United States Holocaust Memorial Museum, "Book Burning."

162 *"fire oaths"*: United States Holocaust Memorial Museum, "Book Burning."

162 *Earlier that week*: Rydell, *Book Thieves*, 6.

162 *By 11:00 p.m. on May 10*: Rydell, *Book Thieves*, 10.

162 *"Where they burn"*: United States Holocaust Memorial Museum, "Book Burning."

162 *impounded the more than ten thousand*: Rydell, *Book Thieves*, 12.

162–63 *Friedenthal had led three departments*: Sächsische Akademie der Wissenshaften zu Leipzig, "Friedenthal, Hans Wilhelm Carl," accessed August 6, 2018, http://drw.saw-leipzig.de/30288/.

163 *Center for Anthropology*: This English name is a very rough translation, as it appears that Friedenthal coined the terms used in the name of his Arbeitsstätte für Menschheitskunde. Translation assistance by Lydia Zoells.

163 *the softness of body hair*: Magnus Hirschfeld Society, "Institut für Sexualwissenschaft (1919–1933)," accessed August 5, 2018, https://magnus-hirschfeld.de/institut/theorie-praxis/zwischenstufen-2-sonstiger-koerperlicher-eigenschaften/.

163 *how human and nonhuman*: Hans Friedenthal, *Tierhaaratlas* (Jena, Germany: G. Fischer, 1911), http://digitalcommons.ohsu.edu/primate/9/.

163 *In 1926 he wrote*: Sigmund Feist, "Are the Jews a Race?," in *Jews and Race: Writings on Identity and Difference, 1880–1940*, ed. Mitchell Bryan Hart (Waltham, MA: Brandeis University Press, 2011), 87.

163 *his family had converted from Judaism*: Martha Friedenthal Haase, "Introduction to the Transaction Edition: Richard Friedenthal and the Story of His Book on the 'German Jupiter,'" in Richard Friedenthal, *Goethe: His Life and Times* (London: Routledge, 2017).

163 *forced out of the University of Berlin*: Sächsische Akademie, "Friedenthal."

163–64 *he sold to a London auction house*: Carolyn Marvin, "The Body of the Text: Literacy's Corporeal Constant," *The Quarterly Journal of Speech* 80, no. 2 (May 1994): 134.

164 *World War I had hit*: Haase, "Introduction."

164 *from the library of a formerly prosperous*: George Bodmer, "A.S.W. Rosenbach: Dealer and Collector," *The Lion and the Unicorn* 22, no. 3 (1998): 277–88.

164 *his adult children*: Haase, "Introduction."

164 *Richard did go*: "Richard Friedenthal, an Author and Head of West German P.E.N.," *The New York Times*, October 22, 1979, accessed July 30, 2018, https://www.nytimes.com/1979/10/22/archives/richard-friedenthal-an-author-and-head-of-west-german-pen.html/.

164 *facing deportation by the Nazis when he killed himself*: Sächsische Akademie, "Friedenthal."

164 *"speculations about"*: Ruth Franklin, *A Thousand Darknesses: Lies and Truth in Holocaust Fiction* (New York: Oxford University Press, 2011), 40–41.

166 *"Dieses Buch wurde"*: Stanford Medicine Lane Medical Library, "Bernardi Siegfried Albini . . . ," accessed October 29, 2018, https://lmldb.stanford.edu/cgi-bin/Pwebrecon.cgi?DB=local&Search_Arg=0359+L32560&Search_Code=CMD*&CNT=10&v2=1/.

166 *A stamped message inside*: Lane Medical Library, "Albini."

166 *"This is one item"*: Drew Bourn, interview with the author, January 20, 2016.

167 *six human skin volumes*: Paul Kersten, "Bucheinbände in Menschenhaut," *Zeitschrift für Bücherfreunde* 8 (1910): 263–64.

167 *"I was the first"*: "Ich bin in Deutschland wohl der erste gewesen, der-im Jahre 1910—den Auftrag erhielt, Bücher in Menschcnhaut zu binden, die ich von einer bekannten Mediziner und Forscher auf dem Gebiete der Haut und der Haare des Menschen und der Säugetiere erhielt, und die ich selbst gerben ließ. Ich darf wohl deshalb als kompetent betrachtet werden, Menschenleder in seinem Aussehen, in

seinen Eigenschaften und in seiner Verarbeitung genau zu kennen und das, was bisher von andern über Menschenleder geschrieben wurde, richtigzustellen." Translation by James Pasternak. Kersten, "Bucheinbände in Menschenhaut": 263–64.

167 *Well respected for his artistry*: Ernst Collin, *Paul Kersten* (Berlin: Corvinus-Antiquariat Ernst Collin G.M.B.H. Verlag, 1925), 12.

167 *He objected to the Nazis' impact*: Helma Schaefer, "Paul Kersten. Wiederentdeckung eines vergessenen Buchbinders," *MDE-Rundbrief: Mitteilungsblatt der Meister der Einbandkunst, MDE-Studienhefte* 2 (2015): 31. Translation by Peter Verheyen.

168 *haunting photograph of Hans Friedenthal*: Landesarchiv Berlin, "Friedenthal, Hans Prof. Dr. med. (geb. 09.07.1870 in Schetnig bei Breslau-gest. 15.08.1942 in Berlin); Anthropologe," accessed July 30, 2018, http://www.landesarchiv-berlin-bilddatenbank.de/hida4web-LAB/view?docId=obj5162783.xml;query=friedenthal;brand=default;doc.style=standardview;blockId=obj%205162783d5033ie2;startDoc=1/.

169 *Hundreds of books*: American Library Association Office for Intellectual Freedom, "Top 10 Most Challenged Books of 2017: Resources & Graphics," accessed August 13, 2018, http://www.ala.org/advocacy/bbooks/NLW-Top10/.

169 *the Harry Potter series*: United States Holocaust Memorial Museum, "Book Burning."

170 *first edition of Pernkopf's*: Sabine Hildebrandt, "How the Pernkopf Controversy Facilitated a Historical and Ethical Analysis of the Anatomical Sciences in Austria and Germany: A Recommendation for the Continued Use of the Pernkopf Atlas," *Clinical Anatomy* 19 (2006): 91.

170 *Scholars researching Pernkopf's*: Hildebrandt, "Pernkopf Controversy," 93.

171 *I was grossly mistaken*: For an excellent primer on Nazi book plunder, see Rydell, *Book Thieves*.

171–72 *tens of millions of books*: Rydell, *Book Thieves*, x.

172 *They repurposed collections*: Rydell, *Book Thieves*, 23.

172 *They planned to form research institutions*: Rydell, *Book Thieves*, 105.

172 *book collecting also conferred status*: Rydell, *Book Thieves*, 62–63.

172 *Heinrich Himmler's penchant*: Rydell, *Book Thieves*, 67–70.

172 *erased or cut out ownership marks*: Rydell, *Book Thieves*, 18.

172 *Other librarians heroically smuggled*: Rydell, *Book Thieves*, 212–13.

172 *Detlef Bockenkamm and Sebastian Finsterwalder*: Rydell, *Book Thieves*, 24.

172 *Their work is not as well supported*: Rydell, *Book Thieves*, 26.

172 *found one book owned by Richard Friedenthal*: Looted Cultural Assets, "Provenienzhinweis: 50 / 5004 (Friedenthal, Richard), Von Hand: Widmung: Allgemein; 'Dem Freunde Dr. Richard Friedenthal Berlin, Dezember 1931 Richard Billinger,'" accessed July 26, 2018, http://lootedculturalassets.de/index.php/Detail/Object/Show/object_id/18270/.

172–73 *another written by Hans Friedenthal*: Looted Cultural Assets, "Exemplar: G45 / 2224, He 39 2.Ex.: Menschheitskunde (1927)," accessed July 26, 2018, http://lootedculturalassets.de/index.php/Detail/Object/Show/object_id/5965/.

173 *Oskar Hein who was murdered*: "Otto Suschny," *Centropa*, accessed July 26, 2018, http://www.centropa.org/de/biography/otto-suschny/.

173 *"These books are like ghosts"*: Rydell, *Book Thieves*, 27.

173 *"the Singing Forest"*: Rydell, *Book Thieves*, 36.

173 *whose legacy the Nazis*: Rydell, *Book Thieves*, 50.

174 *a film*: United States Holocaust Memorial Museum, "German Civilians Visit Buchenwald," accessed July 27, 2018, https://collections.ushmm.org/search /catalog/irn1000201/.

174 *under orders from the American military*: Patricia Heberer Rice, interview with the author, August 2, 2018.

174 *Ilse Koch*: Ruth Franklin, "The READ: How Do We Understand the Holocaust?," *The New Republic*, September 21, 2010, accessed August 11, 2018, https://newrepublic .com/article/77846/the-read-how-do-we-understand-the-holocaust/.

175 *These allegations came up at her trial*: Harry Stein, "Stimmt es, dass die SS im KZ Buchenwald Lampenschirme aus Menschenhaut anfertigen ließ?," Buchenwald and Mittelbau-Dora Memorials Foundation, accessed July 24, 2018, https:// www.buchenwald.de/en/1132.

175 *credible witness testimony*: Stein, "Buchenwald Lampenschirme."

175 *was likely destroyed*: Stein, "Buchenwald Lampenschirme."

175 *Koch's house was searched again in 1943*: Stein, "Buchenwald Lampenschirme."

175 *it disappeared*: Stein, "Buchenwald Lampenschirme."

175 *clear that the lamp was made from animal skin*: Patricia Heberer Rice, interview with the author, August 2, 2018.

175 *those shrunken heads*: Nuremberg Trials Project, "Pohl Case (USA v. Oswald Pohl et al. 1947)," accessed July 15, 2018, http://nuremberg.law.harvard.edu /transcripts/5-transcript-for-nmt-4-pohl-case/.

175 *Some of the human skin items entered into evidence*: Stein, "Buchenwald Lampenschirme."

176 *displayed a third lamp*: Stein, "Buchenwald Lampenschirme."

176 *American serial killer Ed Gein*: Cuskelly, *Original Skin*, 159.

176 *Mark Jacobson's book*: Mark Jacobson, *The Lampshade: A Holocaust Detective Story from Buchenwald to New Orleans* (New York: Simon & Schuster, 2010), 340.

176 *In a subsequent documentary . . . a lab retested*: Steven Hoggard, *Human Lampshade: A Holocaust Mystery* (National Geographic Television, 2012) on Netflix, http://www.imdb.com/title/tt2431232/.

177 *"It's tricky because"*: Patricia Heberer Rice, interview with the author, August 2, 2018.

179 *"When we found out it wasn't real"*: Anonymous, interview with the author, August 14, 2019.

179 We Were in Auschwitz: Ruth Franklin, *A Thousand Darknesses: Lies and Truth in Holocaust Fiction* (New York: Oxford University Press, 2011), 23–26.

179 *"another in the black leather"*: Franklin, "The READ."

179 *"A final copy"*: Franklin, "The READ."

180 *Girs had encountered*: Barbara Girs, interview with the author, May 18, 2019.

180 *three thousand copies printed by the F. Bruckmann printing company*: Barbara Girs, interview with the author, May 18, 2019.

180 *"Salon Bruckmann"*: Katrin Hillgruber, "San Bruckmann: Die Unselige Freitagsgesellschaft," Der Tagesspiegel, October 1, 2010, accessed November 23, 2019, https://www.tagesspiegel.de/kultur/literatur/salon-bruckmann-die-unselige -freitagsgesellschaft/1660844.html.

181 *coerced writers, professors*: Rydell, *Book Thieves*, 13.

181 *Nazi focus on biology*: Robert N. Proctor, "Nazi Doctors, Racial Medicine, and Human Experimentation," in *The Nazi Doctors and the Nuremberg Code*, ed.

George J. Annas and Michael A. Grodin (New York: Oxford University Press, 1992), 19.

181 *physicians rose to become the heads*: Proctor, "Nazi Doctors," 27–28.

181 *excruciating deaths*: Telford Taylor, "Opening Statement of the Prosecution December 9, 1946," in *The Nazi Doctors and the Nuremberg Code*, ed. George J. Annas and Michael A. Grodin (New York: Oxford University Press, 1992), 70.

181 *The Doctors' Trial*: George J. Annas and Michael A. Grodin, introduction to *The Nazi Doctors and the Nuremberg Code*, ed. George J. Annas and Michael A. Grodin (New York: Oxford University Press, 1992), 4.

181 *"perverts"*: Taylor, "Opening Statement," 68.

182 *"In the tyranny"*: Taylor, "Opening Statement," 89.

182 *American doctors cited standards*: Michael A. Grodin, "Historical Origins of the Nuremberg Code," in *The Nazi Doctors and the Nuremberg Code*, ed. George J. Annas and Michael A. Grodin (New York: Oxford University Press, 1992), 134.

182 *Other ideals*: Grodin, "Historical Origins," 123–24.

182 *Ironically, the strongest code*: Sharon Perley et al., "The Nuremberg Code: An International Overview," in *The Nazi Doctors and the Nuremberg Code*, ed. George J. Annas and Michael A. Grodin (New York: Oxford University Press, 1992), 150–51.

182 *dictating a standard*: Grodin, "Historical Origins," 121.

183 *"The voluntary"*: George J. Annas and Michael A. Grodin, eds. *The Nazi Doctors and the Nuremberg Code* (New York: Oxford University Press, 1992), 2.

183 *the delineation between patient*: Perley, "The Nuremberg Code," 159–60.

183 *"The Nuremberg Code's response"*: George J. Annas and Michael A. Grodin, "Where Do We Go from Here?," in *The Nazi Doctors and the Nuremberg Code*, ed. George J. Annas and Michael A. Grodin (New York: Oxford University Press, 1992), 307–308.

11. MY CORPSE, MY CHOICE

185 *"My body is my journal"*: Charles Hamm, interview with the author, October 13, 2015.

186 *"You know"*: Charles Hamm, interview with the author, October 13, 2015.

187 *An Amsterdam-based outfit*: Walls and Skin, "Preserve Your Tattoos," accessed June 30, 2018, http://www.wallsandskin.com/preserveyourtattoos/.

187 *supermodel Kate Moss*: "Kate Moss and the £1million Lucien Freud Tattoo," *The Telegraph*, November 18, 2012, accessed June 30, 2018, https://www.telegraph.co.uk/news/celebritynews/9686095/Kate-Moss-and-the-1million-Lucian-Freud-tattoo.html.

188 *"My skin belongs"*: Harry Low, "The Man Who Sold His Back to An Art Dealer," *BBC News*, February 1, 2017, accessed June 30, 2018, https://www.bbc.com/news/magazine-38601603.

188 *"Can I tell you"*: Charles Hamm, interview with the author, October 13, 2015.

189 *Autopsies and cremation*: Tanya Marsh, e-mail to the author, November 2, 2018.

189 *I read a newspaper article*: "Dead Saskatoon Tattoo Artist Gets Skin Preserved to Honour His Work," *The Globe and Mail*, November 14, 2018, https://www.theglobeandmail.com/canada/article-dead-saskatoon-tattoo-artist-gets-skin-preserved-to-honour-his-work/.

189 *the NAPSA nonprofit had folded*: Kyle Sherwood, interview with the author, November 19, 2018.

189 *"It'd be a shame"*: Kyle Sherwood, interview with the author, November 19, 2018.

190 *"We do a little bit"*: Kyle Sherwood, interview with the author, November 19, 2018.

190 *The Mütter Museum's FAQ*: The Mütter Museum of The College of Physicians of Philadelphia, "FAQ," accessed November 23, 2019, http://muttermuseum.org/about/faq/

190 *2018 donation*: The Mütter Museum of The College of Physicians of Philadelphia, "News of a Rare Donation to the Mütter Museum," May 14, 2018, accessed November 23, 2019, http://muttermuseum.org/news/rare-donation-orzel-FOP/.

190 *"Not liking it"*: Kyle Sherwood, interview with the author, November 19, 2018.

191 *"If I had a [human] skull"*: Tanya Marsh, interview with the author, September 8, 2017.

191 *a corpse is neither a person*: Tanya Marsh, *The Law of Human Remains* (Tucson, AZ: Lawyers & Judges Publishing Company, 2018), ix–x.

191 *Native American Graves*: Marsh, *Law of Human Remains*, 20.

192 *"blazingly idiosyncratic"*: Marsh, *Law of Human Remains*, 42.

192 *"As a society"*: Tanya Marsh, interview with the author, September 8, 2017.

192 *had laws against the disposal*: Stephen F. Clarke, "Law Library of Congress United Kingdom Repatriation of Historic Human Remains," July 2009, accessed June 20, 2018, https://www.loc.gov/law/help/repatriation-human-remains/repatriation-human-remains.pdf, 2.

193 *More than sixty thousand human remains*: Hedley Swain, "Dealings with the Dead: A Personal Consideration of the Ongoing Human Remains Debate," in *Curating Human Remains: Caring for the Dead in the United Kingdom*, ed. Myra Giesen (Suffolk, U.K.: The Boydell Press, 2013), 25.

193 *"through the application of skill"*: Clarke, "United Kingdom Repatriation," 3.

193 *Most of the human remains in museums*: Clarke, "United Kingdom Repatriation," 5.

194 *The Human Tissue Act (HTA) of 2004*: Human Tissue Authority, "List of Materials Considered to Be 'Relevant Material' Under the Human Tissue Act 2004," updated May 2014, accessed June 26, 2018, https://www.hta.gov.uk/policies/list-materials-considered-be-%E2%80%98relevant-material%E2%80%99-under-human-tissue-act-2004/.

194 *The HTA requires*: Human Tissue Authority, "Public Display," accessed June 26, 2018, https://www.hta.gov.uk/regulated-sectors/public-display.

194 *has even more restrictive laws than the U.K.*: Jennifer Sharp and Mark A. Hall, "Tethering Time and Tide? Human Remains Guidance and Legislation for Scottish Museums," in *Curating Human Remains: Caring for the Dead in the United Kingdom*, ed. Myra Giesen (Suffolk, U.K.: The Boydell Press, 2013), 67.

194 *Under Scots law*: Museums Galleries Scotland. *Guideline for the Care of Human Remains in Scottish Museum Collections* (Edinburgh: Museums Galleries Scotland, 2011), accessed June 19, 2018, https://www.museumsgalleriesscotland.org.uk/media/1089/guidelines-for-the-care-of-human-remains-in-scottish-museum-collections.pdf, 5.

194 *granted permanent exceptions*: Sharp, "Tethering Time," 67.

195 *the Field Museum in Chicago*: Te Herekiekie Herewini, "The Museum of New Zealand Te Papa Tongarewa (Te Papa) and the Repatriation of Kōiwi Tangata

(Mäori and Moriori Skeletal Remains) and Toi Moko (Mummified Maori Tattooed Heads)," *International Journal of Cultural Property* 15 (2008): 406.

195 *Some smaller English museums repatriated*: Herewini, "Te Papa," 406.

195 *the British Museum*: Liz White, "The Impact and Effectiveness of the *Human Tissue Act 2004* and the *Guidance for the Care of Human Remains in Museums* in England," in *Curating Human Remains: Caring for the Dead in the United Kingdom*, ed. Myra Giesen (Suffolk, U.K.: The Boydell Press, 2013), 50.

195 *Some small museums in Scotland*: Betsy Inlow, "Cultural Diversity and Inter-Cultural Cooperation: The Life of Horatio Gordon Robley," Scottish Museums Federation, September 12, 2017, accessed July 2, 2018, https://scottishmuseumsfederation .wordpress.com/2017/09/12/cultural-diversity-and-inter-cultural-cooperation-the -life-of-horatio-gordon-robley/.

195 *When the mayor of Rouen*: Laurent Carpentier, "French Museums Face a Cultural Change over Restitution of Colonial Objects," *The Guardian*, November 3, 2014, accessed June 26, 2018, https://www.theguardian.com/world/2014/nov /03/france-museums-restitution-colonial-objects/.

195 *Later, France passed a law*: "Restitution par la France des têtes maories," *Sénat*, June 29, 2009, accessed June 28, 2018, http://www.senat.fr/seances/s200906 /s20090629/s20090629003.html#section293/.

195 *Article 16 of the French Civil Code*: "Article 16," *Codes et Lois*, February 4, 2012, accessed June 28, 2018, https://www.codes-et-lois.fr/code-civil/article-16/.

195 *"any attack on the integrity"*: "Toute atteinte à l'intégrité du cadavre, par quelque moyen que ce soit, est punie d'un an d'emprisonnement et de 15 euros d'amende." Translation by the author. "Article 225–17," *Legifrance*, December 19, 2008, accessed June 28, 2018, https://www.legifrance.gouv.fr/affichCodeArticle.do?idArticle=LEGIARTI000019 983162&cidTexte=LEGITEXT000006070719&dateTexte=20110827.

196 *everywhere worldwide but France*: Charles Hamm, interview with the author, October 13, 2015.

12. THE FRENCH CONNECTION

198 *"sur peau humaine"*: BnF Archives et Manuscrits, "Latin 16268," Bibliothèque nationale de France, https://archivesetmanuscrits.bnf.fr/ark:/12148/cc76740q.

198 *"Abbot Rive alleged"*: "L'abbé Rive a prétendu que ce vélin était de peau de femme. Je pense au contraire qu'il est de peau d'agneau d'irlande mort-né." Translation by the author. BnF Archives et Manuscrits, "Latin 16265," Bibliothèque nationale de France, https://archivesetmanuscrits.bnf.fr/ark:/12148/cc767376.

198 *The final Bible*: BnF Archives et Manuscrits, "Latin 16542," Bibliothèque nationale de France, https://archivesetmanuscrits.bnf.fr/ark:/12148/cc76973d.

199 *In the 1830s,* l'Enfer: Bibliothèque nationale de France, *L'Enfer de la bibliothèque: Éros au secret* (Paris: Bibliothèque nationale de France, 2007), 2, http://www.bnf .fr/documents/dp_enfer.pdf.

200 *What of the rumors about Abbot Jacques Delille*: Ernest de Crauzat, *La reliure française de 1900 à 1925* (Paris: René Kieffer, 1932), 137–39.

200 *Or Verlaine's 1897 book of poetry*: Crauzat, *Reliure française*, 146.

200 *"If we had the power"*: "Aurions-nous le don de traverser les murs et les toits comme don Zombullo du *Diable boiteux*, de nous introduire subrepticement

chez les bibliophiles et de fouiller dans leur bibliothèques, que nous trouverions certainement quelques autres spécimens. Mais combien? Nous n'atteindrions certainement pas la cinquantaine." Translation by the author. Crauzat, *Reliure française*, 149.

201 *"When, at length"*: Edgar Allan Poe, *Tales of Mystery and Imagination* (Mineola, NY: Calla Editions, 2008), 310–11.

202 *"I stay at your entire disposal"*: Frédérick Coxe, e-mail to the author, June 7, 2018.

202 *"Those books make"*: Frédérick Coxe, e-mail to the author, June 11, 2018.

203 *"If not, nevermind"*: Frédérick Coxe, e-mail to the author, June 11, 2018.

203 *"Think about a book on demonology"*: Sébastien Vatinel, e-mail to the author, June 13, 2018.

203 *"The human skin books"*: Sébastien Vatinel, e-mail to the author, June 13, 2018.

204 *"delightfully rare and beautiful"*: Madeleine Le Despencer, e-mail to the author, June 9, 2018.

205–206 *made from pigskin*: Sébastien Vatinel, "Le triple vocabulaire infernal," *Les portes sombres*, accessed November 3, 2018, https://lesportessombres.fr /catalogue/blocquel-le-triple-vocabulaire-infernal/.

206 *"The scientific truth takes"*: Sébastien Vatinel, e-mail to the author, July 4, 2018.

206 The Gold-Bug *was Poe's big break*: Tasha Brandstatter, "The Gold-Bug: The Most Mysterious Edgar Allan Poe Story You've Never Heard Of," *Book Riot*, November 17, 2017, accessed July 5, 2018, https://bookriot.com/2017/11/17/the-gold-bug -edgar-allan-poe/. According to CPI Inflation Calculator (https://www.official data.org/1843-dollars-in-2017), the one hundred dollars Poe won in 1843 would be equivalent to winning $3,312.43 in 2017.

207 *Charles Erskine Scott Wood*: Tim Barnes, "C.E.S. Wood (1852–1944)," in *Oregon Encyclopedia*, March 17, 2018, accessed July 6, 2018, https://oregonencyclopedia .org/articles/c_e_s_wood/#.WoALH6llBAY/.

207 *"Dear John"*: "Poe's Gold-Bug Perhaps in Human Skin," *Live Auctioneers*, updated August 11, 2016, accessed July 5, 2018, https://www.liveauctioneers.com/item /46790564_poe-s-gold-bug-perhaps-in-human-skin/.

207 *Coxe believes that "John"*: Frédérick Coxe, e-mail to the author, July 9, 2018.

207 *our team has confirmed scientifically*: "'Pour en finir' avec les reliures en peau humaine? Epilogue," *Bibliophilie*, July 9, 2018, accessed November 3, 2018, http:// bibliophilie.com/pour-en-finir-avec-les-reliures-en-peau-humaine-epilogue/.

207 *"The purpose is to create"*: Frédérick Coxe, e-mail with the author, July 4, 2018.

208 *"A leader in health education"*: Lawrence K. Altman, "Dr. Russell Lee, 86, Physician; A Pioneer in Group Practice," *The New York Times*, January 29, 1982, accessed July 9, 2018, https://www.nytimes.com/1982/01/29/obituaries/dr-russell -lee-86-physician-a-pioneer-in-group-practice.html/.

208 *He was a beloved clinician*: Claire Norman, "In Memoriam: Peter Lee, 93," *USC News*, August 11, 2016, accessed July 9, 2018, https://news.usc.edu/105240/in -memoriam-peter-lee-93/.

209 *a healthcare adviser in the Obama administration*: Covered California, "Peter V. Lee, Executive Director," accessed November 1, 2018, https://hbex.coveredca .com/executive/.

EPILOGUE: HUMANE ANATOMY

214 *a viable organ donor*: U.S. Department of Health & Human Services, "Organ Donation FAQs," accessed November 1, 2018, https://www.organdonor.gov/about /facts-terms/donation-faqs.html.

214 *patients needing an organ transplant*: The donor list had more than 117,000 people on it as of July 2017. See U.S. Department of Health & Human Services, "Organ Donation FAQs."

214 *twenty dying each day*: United Network for Organ Sharing, "Data," accessed November 1, 2018, https://unos.org/data/.

214 *an opt-in system*: U.S. Department of Health & Human Services, "Organ Donation FAQs."

214 *At USC, you have to die*: University of Southern California Anatomical Gift Program, "Frequently Asked Questions," accessed November 1, 2018, https://agp .usc.edu/frequently-asked-questions/.

215 *risk their health embalming me*: Because of formaldehyde exposure, embalmers have increased risk of cancer (see Judy Walrath and Joseph F. Fraumeni Jr., "Cancer and Other Causes of Death Among Embalmers," *Cancer Research* 44, no. 10 (1984): 4638–41) and potentially ALS (see Mandy Oaklander, "Why Funeral Directors May Be at Higher Risk for ALS," *Time*, July 14, 2015, http://time.com /3956241/funeral-directors-als/).

215 *death-positive movement*: For more, see http://www.orderofthegooddeath.com/.

215 *Death Salons*: For more, see https://deathsalon.org/.

218 *"People always ask"*: Michael Habib, interview with the author, October 17, 2017.

218 *"You get a big cup of coffee"*: Alie Ward, "3-Paleontology with Michael Habib," *Ologies* podcast, October 5, 2017, https://www.alieward.com/ologies/2017/10/5 /3-paleontology-with-michael-habib/.

219 *Alodia Girma said*: Alodia Girma, interview with the author, December 14, 2017.

219 *"Yes, this is a person"*: Alodia Girma, interview with the author, December 14, 2017.

220 *"I think we talked"*: Alodia Girma, interview with the author, December 14, 2017.

220 *In a 2018* Academic Medicine *commentary*: Anne M. Dohrenwend, "Defining Empathy to Better Teach, Measure, and Understand Its Impact," *Academic Medicine*, August 21, 2018 (epub ahead of print).

220 *"Empathy is a conscious"*: Dohrenwend, "Defining Empathy."

221 *"almost articulated fear"*: Dohrenwend, "Defining Empathy."

221 *Diabetics with empathetic doctors*: Mohammadreza Hojat et al., "Physicians' Empathy and Clinical Outcomes for Diabetic Patients," *Academic Medicine* 86, no. 3 (March 2011): 359–64.

221 *decreases malpractice lawsuits*: Kay Kraus and Miriam E. Cameron, "Communication and Malpractice Lawsuits," *Journal of Professional Nursing* 20, no. 1 (January–February 2004): 3.

221 *result patterns are similar worldwide*: Mohammadreza Hojat, *Empathy in Patient Care: Antecedents, Development, Measurement, and Outcomes* (New York: Springer, 2007), 111.

221 *literature and art*: Hojat, *Empathy in Patient Care*, 89.

222 *empathy drops precipitously*: Susan Rosenthal et al., "Humanism at Heart: Preserving Empathy in Third-Year Medical Students," *Academic Medicine* 86 (2011): 350–51.

222 *report the lowest satisfaction*: Liselotte N. Dyrbye et al., "Physician Satisfaction and Burnout at Different Career Stages," *Mayo Clinic Proceedings* 88, no. 12 (2013): 1360–61.

222 *young doctors cope*: Christina Maslach et al., "Job Burnout," *Annual Review of Psychology* 52 (2001): 403.

223 *on an auctioneer's slab in Kentucky*: Guy Hinsdale, "A Description of the Skeleton of the American Giant, with a Note on the Relation of Acromegaly and Giantism," *Transactions of the College of Physicians of Philadelphia*, Third Series, vol. 20 (1898): 151, https://archive.org/details/s3transactionsstud2ocoll/.

224 *Usually caused by benign brain tumors*: U.S. National Library of Medicine, "Acromegaly," MedlinePlus, updated October 1, 2018, https://medlineplus.gov/ency/article/000321.htm.

225 *"Oh my god, I was so scared"*: Catherine Curran, interview with the author, October 13, 2017.

226–27 *"I think everything"*: Catherine Curran, interview with the author, October 13, 2017.

227 *"Imagine yourself going in"*: Catherine Curran, interview with the author, October 13, 2017.

ACKNOWLEDGMENTS

I am forever grateful to all the people who helped midwife this strange little book into the world. Queen among them is my agent, Anna Sproul-Latimer, who believed in me when I was just a morbid librarian with a dream. Amanda Moon's rigorous eye tortured me just enough to make this book the best it could be, and her sweet enthusiasm always guided me gently back from the edge; it was an honor working with her. Thanks to Julia Ringo and the whole team at Farrar, Straus and Giroux for somehow letting me join the pantheon of my favorite writers at this storied house; I hope I do you proud.

To the amazing librarians and museum curators who allowed me to skulk around their stacks and inboxes, I am so thankful. Special thanks to those word workers who helped me along the way, including James Pasternak for his German assistance, Gemma Angel, Robert Johnson, Deborah Harkness, Peter Verheyen, Jesse Meyer at Pergamena, and Tanya Marsh for serving as my "corpse law" attorney on (unpaid) retainer. My dear friend Joe Decarolis came through with a Hail Mary archives assist that was so unexpected and amazing. My deepest gratitude to Jillian Tullis and TaRosa Jacobs for their thoughtful reads. It takes a village of morbid weirdos.

Thanks to the boards who saw my absurd-sounding grant proposals to travel the world looking for human skin books and chose to fund me anyway, including the boards of USC's Zumberge Individual Fund Award, the MLGSCA Professional Development Award, and the Wood Institute for the History of Medicine Travel Grant. Thanks to those colleagues at the University of Southern California who supported me throughout the research and writing of this book.

My undying love goes to the fine people of the death-positive movement, in particular Caitlin Doughty, whose judgment and sensitivity are beyond compare, and without whom I would have never had such amazing opportunities and experiences. Deepest thanks to all those in the Order of the Good Death—especially Sarah Chavez, Louise Hung, Elizabeth Harper, Landis Blair, Colin Dickey, and Paul Koudounaris—who are the most cooperative, amazing group of thinkers and friends. A special thanks goes to Lindsey Fitzharris, my number-one morbid cheerleader, who has championed this book so generously and whose friendship means the world to me. A thank-you also to Erik Larson for the best pep talk of all time.

Thank you to the Anthropodermic Book Project—Anna Dhody, Richard Hark, and Daniel Kirby—for your fine work; it is a pleasure doing science with you. Thanks also to Rebecca Michaelson for her assistance in building our team's database.

Trying to write a book while working full-time and mothering a baby really does take a village, and mine was so large it might be considered a city outright. Thanks to the Hazelcare squad of Aviva and Ben Rosenbloom, Melissa Balick, Aradenia Aguilar, Nadia and Siena Thomas, and the ladies of MFG. Thanks to the Megancare cabal of Cindy Scherban, Angela DiBlasi, Megan Klammer, Karin Saric, AJ Hawkins, Jenn Tran, Corinne Elicone, and Racelle Rosett. Thanks to Lori Snyder and the writers of Splendid Mola, cheese, book club members past and present, and all my friends who inspire me with their lives and art, or have swooped in with a well-timed word of encouragement or commiseration over a beer.

For Jonathan Gold: it kills me that you'll never see this book, but I hope you knew how honored I was to be your friend.

To my husband, Etan Rosenbloom, how can I even begin to enumerate the ways, great and small, that you stepped up for our family to make this book come into being? You are the best person I have ever known, *the end*. And to Hazel Erev Rosenbloom, my unwitting coauthor: I know now that birthing a book and a baby at the same time wasn't the wisest choice a mama could make, but I appreciate your being such a cute good sport about it. The book may have gotten done a lot quicker without you on the scene, but it wouldn't have been half as much fun. Etan and Hazel, I look forward to devoting my full attention to you again.

Last, for all of those whose histories I uncovered—and for the countless others whose tales might never be revealed—I hope I did your stories justice in this book.

Index

academia, *see* medical schools; *specific universities*
Academic Medicine, 220
Acres of Books, 106
acromegaly, 225, 227
Act of Parliament (1752), 125, 137
adipocere bodies, 63
Africa, 95, 104
Alaska, 29, 30, 74
Albinus, Bernhard Siegfried, *De sede et caussa coloris Aethiopum et caeterorum hominum*, 165
American Journal of the Medical Sciences, The, 50
American Medical Association, 57, 182
American Revolution, 11, 12, 92, 95–96
ammonia, 72
amputation, 61
anatomical pathology, 44
anatomy, 8, 10–11, 43, 44–45, 52, 59–64, 80, 110–13, 211–27; Burke and Hare murders, 131–45; cadaver procurement norms and ethics, 59–65, 130, 131–45, 169–71; French Revolution-era, 43–46; laws, 137–44; murderabilia, 123–30; Pernkopf's *Atlas*, 169–72; photography, 127; riots, 143–44; whole body donation, 213–23; *see also* cadavers; dissection
Anatomy Act, 128, 138–44
ancestry tests, 31–32
animal skins, used for bookbinding, 13–16, 22, 32, 68–77, 167, 198, 206; camel, 97; cow, 13, 16, 22, 101, 198, 176; follicle patterns, 22, 72, 167; horse 46, 97; parchment, 11, 15, 68, 70, 71, 74, 89, 198; rabbit, 71, 181; tanning methods, 68–77

Annas, George, 183
Anonymous, *Le traicté de Peyne: poëme allégorique dédié à Monseigneur et à Madame de Lorraynne*, 229
anthropodermic bibliopegy, *see* human skin books
Anthropodermic Book Project, ix, 9, 10, 12, 33, 65, 168, 177, 178, 181, 190, 201; list of confirmed human skin books, 229–30
anthropodermic books, *see* human skin books
anti-Semitism, 163, 164, 168, 172–83
apprenticeship, 43
Arch Street Bones Project, 64
artisan guilds, 38, 84
association copies, 157
asylum inmates, 49, 156, 187
Attucks, Crispus, 92, 95–98, 110
Attucks, Nancy, 95
Auschwitz, 179
autopsy, 50, 55, 77, 82, 215; as desecration, 189

Baker, Nicholson, *Double Fold: Libraries and the Assault on Paper*, 87
Balsam, Eliza, 124
Bancroft Library, at the University of California, Berkeley, 35–38, 46
Barles, Louis, *Les nouvelles découvertes sur toutes les parties principales de l'homme, et de la femme*, 50, 229
bating, 73
Bechtel, Guy, 202
Belot, Adolphe, *Mademoiselle Giraud, My Wife*, 229

Bentham, Jeremy, 137–38, 144;
  Benthamites, 138
Berlin, 161, 162, 163, 168
Bible, 89, 104, 197, 198
bibliomania, 17, 27, 58, 167
Bibliothèque nationale de France, 42, 53,
  197–99, 201, 206; *Catalog des sciences
  médicales*, 53–55, 230; Richelieu
  Library, 197–99; *see also* France
"A Bill for Regulating Schools of
  Anatomy," 140–41
biocodicology, 14–15, 71
Blacks, 92; abused by White doctors,
  110–13; authors, 104–10; cadavers,
  110–13; free, 105–10; human skin
  books and, 92, 95–113; lynchings,
  110–13; oral tradition, 110; slaves, 95,
  104, 105, 106, 110–11
Bockenkamm, Detlef, 172
body donation, whole, 213–23
Book Farm, 107
bookworms, 100
Borowski, Tadeusz, 179; *Imiona Nurtu*,
  180–81; *We Were in Auschwitz*, 179–80
Boston, 95–96, 104–105, 147, 154
Boston Athenæum, 154–59
Boston Massacre, 95–96
Boston Medical Library, 58
Bouland, Ludovic, 20–22, 28, 86, 89,
  91–93, 109, 158
Bourgeois, Louise, 79–85; folk remedies
  of, 83 and *n*; *Observations*, 80; *Recueil
  des secrets de Louyse Bourgeoise*, 50,
  83, 84, 229
Bourn, Drew, 166, 169
brain tumors, 224, 225, 227
Brandt, Randal, 36–38
Breil, André du, 84
Brenner, Elma, 91–92
British Museum, 195
Brown University, 106*n*, 108; John Hay
  Library, ix
Bruckmann printing company, 180 and *n*
Buchenwald, 173–75
Bunker, Chang and Eng, 3
Burke, William, 131–45, 194

Burke and Hare murders, 131–45; *see also*
  West Port Murders
Burke's Skin Pocket Book, 132–33
burking, 135, 140, 143
Bury St. Edmunds, 118–30

cadavers, 4, 10, 44–45, 52, 59–64;
  Anatomy Act, 138–44; Black,
  110–13; Burke and Hare murders,
  131–45; donor anonymity, 213; humane
  treatment, 211–27; Paris School and,
  44–46; Pernkopf's *Atlas*, 169–72;
  photography, 126; procurement norms
  and ethics, 59–65, 130, 131–45, 169–71;
  Soap Lady, 62–65; tattoo preservation,
  185–92; whole body donation, 213–23;
  see also anatomy; dissection
calfskin, 22, 69, 71, 76, 167, 180
California Rare Book School, 35
Calnan, Christopher, 97 and *n*, 98
camel skin, 97
Cantin, 42–44
Carnegie, Dale, *Lincoln the Unknown*, 103*n*
cellulose, 178
chamber-lye, 72
chamber pot, 67, 72, 75
Chapin, Mrs. H. M., 154
Chaplin, Simon, 127, 128
Chapman, Nathaniel, 57–58
Château de Meudon, 38–40
Chaucer, Geoffrey, 36
chemistry, 29, 43, 201
childbirth, 79–84
cholera, 143
Christianity, 89, 94, 152, 197
chrome tanning method, 68, 70
Cincinnati, 106
Cincinnati Public Library, 106
Civil War, American, 4, 61, 154;
  casualties, 4, 61–62
clinical gaze, 8, 17, 44–46, 60, 62, 84, 126,
  183, 213, 222
clinical medicine, 8, 15–16, 57–58;
  Anatomy Act, 138–44; cadaver
  dissection, 44–46, 59–64; cadaver

procurement norms and ethics, 59–65, 130, 131–45; development of, 8, 33, 43–47, 57–64, 83, 84; empathy, 220–23; importance of object acquisition, 58–59; modern system of, 44–47; Nuremberg Code, 182–83; Paris School, 44–46; whole body donation, 213–23; *see also* doctors

collagen, 14

College of Physicians of Philadelphia, 3–6, 7, 9, 24, 32, 33 and *n*, 36, 37, 52, 55, 62–64, 73, 74, 77, 189–90, 223, 226; *see also* Mütter Museum

colonial life, 57, 95–98, 104–5

Columbus, Christopher, 99–100, 102

Committee of Investigation as to the Dealings of Dr. Knox with the West Port Murders, 137

concentration camps, 173–75; medical experimentation, 181–83

consent, 144–45, 182–83, 185–96; corpses and, 185–96; informed, 182–83; laws on human remains, 144, 182–83, 191–95; Nazism and, 182–83; Nuremberg Code, 182–83; tattoo preservation, 185–92

conservation of books, 9, 15, 22, 29–30, 70, 87, 97, 99, 109, 155

Conté, Nicolas-Jacques, 40

Coralla, Sebastian Carroll Braganza de la, 100–103

Corder, William, 115–30, 132, 158; cremation of, 127, 193; dissection of, 122–23, 126; execution of, 120–24; human skin book, 123–30, 193; murderabilia, 123–30; museum protocol on human remains, 128–29; Red Barn murder, 115–30; skeleton of, 126–28, 193; trial of, 118–20, 125

corpse desecration, 188–91

Countway Library of Medicine, at Harvard University, 22–27, 187

Couper, Robert, *Speculations on the Mode and Appearances of Impregnation in the Human Female*, 50, 229

cowhide, 13, 16, 22, 176; *see also* vellum

Coxe, Frédérick, 202–203, 206, 209

Crauzat, Ernest de, *La reliure française de 1900 à 1925*, 200, 201

Creed, George, 121–23

creepypastas, 17 and *n*

cremation, 186, 188, 193, 215; as desecration, 189

cryptography, 206

Cudmore, George, 124

currency, skin as, 11

Cushing, Stanley, 155–57

d'Agoty, Jacques, 7

Dance of Death, The, ix, 106*n*, 108, 229

Darwin, Charles, 61

death, 16, 18, 211–27; allegedly murderer-derived human skin books, 123–30; Black lynchings, 110–12; Burke and Hare murders, 131–45; in childbirth, 82–83; consent and, 185–96; corpses of murdered women exploited, 90–92; flayed corpses, 121–22; French Revolution, 37–38; masks, 121–23, 124, 125, 132; mementos, 123–30; penalty, 125, 153; Red Barn murder, 115–30; tattoo preservation, 185–92

death positivity, 171, 190, 211–27

Death Salons, 215–16, 226

Deck, Isaiah, 88

Declaration of Independence, 96, 104

Declarations of Helsinki, 183

deerskin, 153

Delille, Abbot Jacques, 200

Delvoye, Wim, 187

depersonalization, 222–23

Deutsche Studentenschaft, 161–62

Dhody, Anna, 32, 64, 190

diabetes, 221

digestive enzymes, 73

digital materials, 17, 156, 157, 158, 204

dissection, 4, 10, 44–45, 52, 59–64, 120, 211–27; Anatomy Act, 138–44; of Black corpses, 110–13; Burke and Hare murders, 131–45; cadaver procurement norms and ethics,

dissection (*cont.*)
  59–65, 130, 131–45, 169–71; of William
  Corder, 122–23, 126; Pernkopf's *Atlas*,
  169–72; photography, 126; whole body
  donation, 213–23; *see also* anatomy;
  cadavers
DNA testing, 14–15, 31–32, 176
Docherty, Mary, 136
doctor bibliophiles, 4, 8, 10, 51; Bouland,
  Ludovic, 20–22, 28, 86, 89, 91–93,
  109, 158; Friedenthal, Hans, 162–69,
  172, 173, 174; Hough, John Stockton,
  50–57; Lee, Russell van Arsdale,
  207–9; Leidy, Joseph, 4, 56–65; Osler,
  William, 58; Watson, Blake, 10
doctors, 4, 8, 10, 15–16, 33, 211–27;
  Anatomy Act, 138–44; Black
  patients abused by, 110–13; Burke
  and Hare murders, 131–45; cadaver
  procurement norms and ethics,
  59–65, 130, 131–45, 169–71; class, 8;
  development of clinical medicine
  and, 8, 33, 43–47, 57–64, 83, 84;
  empathy, 220–23; female, 84–85;
  French Revolution, 42–47; gender
  bias, 84–85; human skin book
  collections of, 4–5, 8, 10–11, 33, 50–65,
  72–77, 84–86; importance of object
  acquisition, 58–59; midwives and,
  79–84; Nazi, 181–83; Nuremberg
  Code, 182–83; patient relationship,
  44, 220–23; portraits of, 126; *see also*
  clinical medicine; *specific doctors*
Dohrenwend, Anne, 220
Donald, 134
Drelincourt, Charles, *De conceptione
  adversaria*, 55, 229
Dube, Liz, 100, 101, 103

Eastlack, Harry, 190n
Eckert, Jack, 22–27, 28
economy, livestock, 71
Edinburgh, 131–45
Egyptian mummies, 88
elephant skin, 33n

Éloge des seins, 200
embalming, 215
Emerson, Ralph Waldo, 154
empathy, 226–27; clinician, 220–23
Encylopædia Britannica, 39
England, 89–92, 95–96, 105, 164; anatomy
  laws, 137–44; Human Tissue Act
  (HTA) law, 194; laws on human
  remains, 191–95; Red Barn murder,
  115–30
Eppendorf Tubes, 7
Étienne, Louis Félix, 41
Euclid, 105
evolution, 13, 14, 32, 163
executed criminals, alleged human skin
  books made from, 123–30, 153–59

Fabricius ab Acquapendente, *De formato
  foetu*, 51
fakes, 33, 92–93, 96–104, 129–30, 201;
  Attucks book, 95–98; provenance
  trap, 98–99; *see also* forgery
Female Lunatic Asylum, 49
Fenno, John, 150, 151, 153, 154
fetal development, 51
fibrodysplasia ossificans progressiva
  (FOP), 190n
Fiddyment, Sarah, 71
Field Museum, Chicago, 195
Finsterwalder, Sebastian, 172, 173
Firestone Library, at Princeton
  University, 85
fish tanning, 74
Fitzharris, Lindsey, 90
flayed corpses, 121–22
Foik, Father Paul, 101–102
Folger Shakespeare Library, 164
folio, 36
follicle patterns, 22, 23–25, 72–73, 92, 97,
  103, 167, 203
forceps, 81
forgery, 16, 96–104, 129–30; *see also* fakes
formaldehyde, 216
Foucault, Michel, *The Birth of the Clinic*,
  44–46

Foundation of the Art and Science of Tattooing, 187

France, 19, 20, 37–38, 53–54, 79–84, 195–96, 197–209; Constitution of 1793, 40–41, 46; human skin books, 37–47, 197–209; laws on human remains, 195–96; Meudon tannery, 38–40; midwives, 79–84; occult books, 202–7; Paris School, 44–46; Revolution-era human skin books, 37–47, 54, 200; *see also* Bibliothèque nationale

Franklin, Benjamin, 96, 105

Franklin, Ruth, 164, 179

Freemasons, 172

Freud, Lucian, 187

Friedenthal, Hans, 162–69, 172, 173, 174; human skin books, 164–69

Friedenthal, Richard, 164

funeral homes, 189

Galen, 82

gallows humor, 126

gangrene, 82

Gates, Henry Louis, 105

gay and trans people, 162, 172

Geddes, Annabel, 90–92

Gein, Ed, 176

gender, 28, 84–86; corpses of murdered women exploited, 90–92; human skin books and, 85–86; sexist attitudes toward women doctors, 84–85

genetics, 14–15, 31–32, 163

Germany, 70, 161–83; bookbinding, 167–68; civilians, 174; Doctor's Trial, 181–82; Holocaust, 164, 173–83; Nazi, 161–83; Nazi doctors, 181–83; post–World War II, 176; Third Reich, 161n

gibbet, 124–25, 137

Gibson, Thomas, aka M.N., 10; *Anatomy Epitomized and Illustrated . . .*, 8–11, 16, 230

gigantism, 223–27

gilding, 55, 100, 153, 179, 206

Girma, Alodia, 219, 220, 223

Girs, Anatol, 179–80

Girs, Barbara, 179–80

gloves, for handling rare books, 21

goatskin, 13, 68, 167

Goebbels, Joseph, 161

Goethe, Johann Wolfgang von, 164, 173–74

Granary Burying Ground, 96

grave robbing, 131, 133–44, 191

Graves, Joseph L., 32

great apes, 13–14

Greece, 82

Grodin, Michael, 183

Grolier Club, 51, 53

Guillemeau, Charles, 81, 82, 83

Guillemeau, Jacques, 81; *De la grossesse et accouchement des femmes*, 80–81

guillotine, 37

Gunn, Alistair, 91

Gutenberg Bible, 89

Guthrie, G. J., 138–39

Gutiérrez, Juan, *Practicarum quaestionum circa leges regias Hispaniae*, 22

Habib, Michael, 216, 218 and n, 222, 223

hair, 163, 177, 194

Hamm, Charles, 185–90, 195–96

hangings, 110–11, 120–21, 133, 173

Hare, William, 131–45

Hark, Richard, 32, 108

Harvard Law School Library, 22

Harvard Library, 9, 13, 19–22, 24–25, 27, 30, 32, 85, 86–88, 89

Hawthorne, Nathaniel, 154

heads, 195; preserved tattooed, 195; shrunken, 174, 175

Heartman (Charles F.) Collection of Material Relating to Negro Culture, 106

Heartman, Charles, 106–9

Heberer Rice, Patricia, 177, 179

Hein, Oskar, 173

Heine, Heinrich, 162

Henry IV, King of France, 81

Hesburgh Library, at the University of Notre Dame, 99–103

Himmler, Heinrich, 172

Hippocrates, 82–83
Hippocratic Oath, 182
Hirschfeld, Magnus, 162
Hitler, Adolf, 168, 180n, 181
Holbein, Hans, *The Dance of Death*, ix, 106n, 108, 229
Holocaust, 164, 173–83
hormonal imbalance, 223–27
horse leather, 46, 97
Horwood, John, 124
Hough, John Stockton, 50–57, 62, 72, 84, 158; human skin book collection of, 50–57, 67, 72–77, 84–86; "Two Cases of Trichiniasis at the Philadelphia Hospital, Blockley," 50
Houghton Library, at Harvard University, 19–22, 27, 30, 32, 85, 86–89, 106
Houssaye, Arsène, 20–21; *Des destinées de l'ame*, 19–22, 26–29, 86, 89, 230
human growth hormone (HGH), 223–25
human skin books, 4–18; age of, 25–26; allegedly made from executed criminals, 123–30, 153–59; allegedly murderer-derived, 123–30; Anatomy Act, 138–44; Blacks and, 92, 95–113; Burke's Skin Pocket Book, 132–33; Corder, 123–30, 193; depersonalization and, 222–23; *Des destinées de l'ame*, 19–22, 26–29, 86, 89; doctor bibliophiles, 4, 8, 10, 51; fakes, 33, 92–93, 96–104, 129–30, 201; follicle patterns, 22–25, 72–73, 92, 97, 103, 167, 203; French, 37–47, 197–209; French Revolution-era, 37–47, 54, 200; Friedenthal, 164–65; gender and, 85–86; list of confirmed books, 229–30; made from dead soldiers, 62; monetary value of, 16, 22, 99, 101, 207; Nazis and, 173–83; peptide mass fingerprinting (PMF) tests on, 13–16, 22, 27, 30–32, 46, 87, 97, 109, 157, 168–69, 181, 203, 205, 207; physician collectors of, 4–5, 8, 10–11, 33, 50–65, 72–77, 84–86; race and, 31–32, 92–93, 95–113; tanning for, 67–77; terminology, 4, 17, 86; Walton, 153–59, 229; Wheatley, 106–10, 229,

230; women's skin used for, 50–57, 67, 72–77, 85–86, 91, 199; *see also specific authors, books, collectors, and libraries*
Human Tissue Act (HTA), 194
Hunt, Henry, 139
Hunt, William, 63
Hunter, John, 127, 128
Hunterian, at the Royal College of Surgeons of England, 127, 193
Huntington Library, Art Museum, and Botanical Gardens, 6–16, 164; Munger Research Center, 6–16

illiteracy, 11
illness, 16, 49–51, 56–57, 143, 151, 223–27
incunabula, 42, 51, 54
Indiana State University, 158
industrialization, 57, 68
influenza, 151–52
insects, 100
Institute of Sexual Studies (Institut für Sexualwissenschaft, or ISS), 162–63
Institut zur Erforschung der Judenfrage, 172
integritatis & corruptionis virginum notis, De, 91–92
Internet, 17, 156
Ireland, 140, 192

Jack the Ripper, 90–91
Jack the Ripper Museum, 91
Jacobson, Mark, *The Lampshade*, 176
Jakob-Krause-Bund, 167
Jefferson, Thomas, 104
Jefferson Scale of Physician Empathy (JSPE), 221–22
Jews, 163, 179; Nazi persecution of, 163, 164, 168, 172–83; suicides, 164
John Hay Library, at Brown University, ix
Johnson, Michael, 95
Joseph, Michael, 108
Joseph the Miller, 134
Juniata College, 22

Keck School of Medicine of USC, 213
Kennedy, John F., 154
Kennedy, Ted, 154, 208–209
Kersten, Paul, 166, 167, 168
Kirby, Daniel, 13, 29–32, 33 and *n*, 46, 54
Knox, Robert, 134–45
Koch, Ilse, 174–75
Koch, Karl-Otto, 175
Koran, 30

l'Admiral, Jan, 165
lampredotto, 69
lampshades, human skin, 174–79
Lancet, The, 140
Lander, Beth, 52, 56, 74
Landesarchiv Berlin, 168
Lane, Bill, 30
Lane Medical Library, 164
lant, 72
laws, 188–96; anatomy, 138–44; corpse
    desecration, 188–91; Human Tissue
    Act (HTA), 194; on human remains,
    138–44, 182–83, 188–96; Native
    American Graves Protection and
    Repatriation Act (NAGPRA), 191–92;
    Nuremberg Code, 182–83
Le Despencer, Madeleine, 204
Lee, Peter, 208, 209, 219
Lee, Russell van Arsdale, 207–9
Leidy, Joseph, 4, 56–65, 112, 135, 158, 217,
    218 and *n*, 223; *An Elementary Treatise
    on Human Anatomy*, 4, 61, 62, 217, 229;
    human skin book collection of, 61–65;
    Mütter American Giant and, 223–27;
    Soap Lady cadaver and, 59–65
libraries, 35–38, 156, 164, 208–9;
    challenged books, 169–71; French,
    42, 53, 197–99; future of research
    libraries, 156–57; list of confirmed
    human skin books in, 229–30; Nazi
    looting of, 171–73; *see also specific
    libraries, librarians, authors, and books*
liming process, 72–73
l'imposture des diables, De, 202
Lincoln, Charles, 150–52, 155–56, 158

Liston, Robert, 133
London, 89–92, 105, 108, 118, 137, 140,
    163, 164, 187, 204
London Dungeon, 90–91
Los Angeles County Medical
    Association, 10
Louis XIII, King of France, 79, 81–82
Louis XV, King of France, 38
Louis XVI, King of France, 38
Low, Peter, 153–54
Luther, Martin, 164
Lynch, Mary, 49–57, 65, 151, 227; books
    made from skin of, 50–57, 67, 72–77,
    85–86

MALDI plate, 13
malpractice lawsuits, 221
Manchester, 140, 143
Manifest Destiny, 16
Mann, Thomas, 161 and *n*
Maori Toi moko, 195
Marie de Bourbon-Montpensier,
    Princess, 82
Marie de Médicis, Queen of France, 79–82
Mark Twain Project, 36
Marsh, Tanya, 191, 192; *The Law of
    Human Remains*, 191
Marten, Ann, 115, 116, 117
Marten, George, 116
Marten, Maria, 115–30
Marten, Thomas, 116, 117, 125
Massachusetts, 95, 104, 147–52; state
    prison, 150–52
mass-market publication, 87
Mass Spectrometry and Proteomics
    Resource Laboratory, 30
McCloskey, Thomas, 56
medical consent, concept of, 144–45
medical education, 42–46, 61, 133–34,
    211–33; body donation for, 214–23;
    empathy, 220–23; laws governing,
    137–44; USC anatomy program,
    211–23; *see also* Paris School; *specific
    universities*
medieval books, 15, 71, 101, 197–98

memoirs, 179–81; Holocaust, 179–80; as
    human skin books, 153–59
Merrifield, Edward, *The Story of the
    Captivity and Rescue from the Indians
    of Luke Swetland*, 11–12, 16, 41
metalwork, 55, 100, 153, 165, 206
Meudon tannery, 38–40
Meyer, Jesse, 69–76
Meyers (Richard E.) & Sons, 70
microfiche, 87, 88
microscope, 57
midwives, 79–84; see also sages-femmes
Milton, John: *Paradise Lost*, 105, 106; *The
    Poetical Works of John Milton*, 124
Mississippi, 107, 108
Monro, Alexander, 132, 133, 134
Montaigne, Michel de, 190
Montgaillard, Abbot Guillaume Honoré
    Rocques de, 39
Montgaillard, Count de, 39
Moors, 99, 100, 102
Mount Moriah Cemetery, 64
Mount Vernon, 154
Moyse's Hall Museum, 124–25, 127, 137,
    193
Mullen's Tannery, 24
mummification, 14, 88, 125
Munger Research Center, at the
    Huntington Library, Art Museum,
    and Botanical Gardens, 6–16
murder, 90–92; allegedly murderer-
    derived human skin books,
    123–30; Burke and Hare murders,
    131–45; corpses of murdered women
    exploited, 90–92; mementos,
    123–30; Red Barn murder, 115–30;
    Whitechapel, 90–91
murderabilia, 123–30
Murrell, Ron, 125, 126
Musée Carnavalet, 40–41, 46
Museum for German History
    (Museum für Deutsche Geschichte),
    176
museum protocol on human remains,
    128–29
Mütter American Giant, 223–27

Mütter Museum, 3–6, 9, 32, 33 and *n*, 36,
    62–65, 190 and *n*, 216, 223–27; see also
    College of Physicians of Philadelphia
Mysteries of the Museum (TV show), 155

nails, 194
Napoleon Bonaparte, 41
Nash, Bob, 60
National Association for the
    Preservation of Skin Art (NAPSA),
    185, 186, 188, 189
National Socialist Physician's League, 181
National Trust for Places of Historic
    Interest or Natural Beauty, 92, 97
Native American Graves Protection and
    Repatriation Act (NAGPRA), 191–92
Native Americans, 11–12, 16, 95, 191;
    claims to human remains, 191–94
Nazis, 4, 161–83; books burnt by, 161–62,
    171; books stolen by, 171–73; doctors,
    181–83; human skin books, 173–83;
    human skin lampshades, 174–79;
    Pernkopf's *Atlas*, 169–72; racial
    policies, 163, 164, 168, 172–73
necrophilia, 28
Needham, Paul, 27–28, 85–89, 109
Nessworthy, Linda, 127
Netflix, 155
Netter's Atlas of Anatomy, 217
New Jersey, 55, 70, 106
New Orleans, 176
newsprint, 87–88
New York, 11, 51, 107
New York Times, The, 158, 208
New Zealand, 195
Norris Medical Library, at University of
    Southern California, 169
Nuremberg, 181–83
Nuremberg Code, 182–83

Obama, Barack, 209
obesity, 215
object acquisition, importance of, 58–59
occult books, 172, 202–207

office de l'église en François, L', 37–41
Old Blockley, *see* Philadelphia General Hospital
Ologies, 218
"ooze" binding, 155; *see also* suede
Opera Joannis Pici Mirandule, 99–103
organ donation, 214
Orléans, Duke of, 39
Orzel, Carol, 190*n*
Osler, William, 58
Ovid, *Metamorphoses*, 24–26

papermaking, 35–36
papyrus, 36, 68
parchment, 11, 15, 68, 70, 71, 74, 89, 198; books, 15; *see also* vellum
Paré, Ambroise, 80
Paris, 38, 40, 44–46, 80, 82, 197, 199
Paris School, 44–46
Paterson, David, 136
Peabody Museum of Archaeology & Ethnology, at Harvard University, 29–30
Pearson, David, *Provenance Research in Book History*, 156–57
peptide mass fingerprinting (PMF), 13–16, 21–22, 27, 30–32, 46, 87, 97, 109, 157, 168–69, 181, 203, 205, 207
Pergamena, 68–77
peritonitis, 82
Pernkopf's *Atlas*, 169–72
Peters, John, 106
Philadelphia, 3, 9, 49, 56–64, 70, 226
Philadelphia General Hospital, 49–52, 55, 56, 75
Philadelphia *Public Ledger*, 63
Philadelphia School of Anatomy, 59
photography, dissection, 126
phrenology, 122–23
phthisis, *see* tuberculosis
pickling brine, 72
Pico della Mirandola, Giovanni, 99–100; *Oration on Human Dignity*, 99
pigskin, 22, 103, 167, 203, 204, 206
pituitary gland, 224

placenta, 82
plague, 14–15
plaster death masks, 121–23, 124, 125
plastic surgery, 186
pocketbooks, 92, 96
Poe, Edgar Allan, *The Gold-Bug*, 201, 202, 203, 206–209
Pollack, John, 52–55
poorhouses, 138, 141
Pope, Alexander, 104
pork, 203; *Trichinae spiralis* in, 49, 56–57
Portland Art Museum, 207
Princeton University, 27, 85–86; Firestone Library, 85
prison, 120–121, 148–59, 187; alleged human skin books made from executed criminals, 153–59; cemetery, 158; concentration camps, 173–75; escapes, 148–49; gaol, 115
Proceedings of the National Academy of Sciences, 71
proteins, 13–15, 29
proteomics, 29
provenance trap, 98–99
Puglia, Alan, 30

quarter-bound books, 53
quarto, 36

rabbit skin, 71, 181
race, 31–32, 92–93, 95–113; Blacks abused by White doctors, 110–13; false claims about, 99–103; human skin books and, 31–32, 92–93, 95–113
rag paper, 35, 87–88, 89
rebinding, 26, 87
Red Barn murder, 115–30
Reich Health Council, 182
Reinking, Rik, 188
relic hunters, 121–30
Renaissance, 40, 99
repatriation of human remains, 191–96
research libraries, future of, 156–57
resurrectionists, 134–44

Richardson, Ruth, 142; *Death, Dissection, and the Destitute*, 142, 144
Richelieu Library, at the Bibliothèque nationale de France, 197–99
Rights of Man, The, 38
rigor mortis, 76
rodents, 101
Rogers, Abner, 155–56
Rome, 82
Rosner, Lisa, *The Anatomy Murders*, 135
roundworm infection, 49
Royal College of Surgeons of Edinburgh, 132, 135, 138, 140, 141; Surgeons' Hall Museums, 132, 194
Royal College of Surgeons of England, 127, 128; Hunterian, 127, 193
Royal Society of Edinburgh, 136
Rugg, George, 100, 102
Rutgers University, 108
Ruysch, Frederick, 165

Sade, Marquise de, *Justine et Juliette*, 199
sages-femmes, 79–84; *see also* midwives
sailors, 187
San Francisco, 203, 207
Sanitary Commission, 61
Sansale, Gayet de, 198–99
Satterlee military hospital, 61–62
SaveMyInk.com, 185, 186, 187
Save My Ink Forever, 189, 191, 192, 196
Schafhirt, Fred, 60
Scheide, William, 85–86
Schomburg, Arthur, 107
Scotland, 192, 194; Burke and Hare murders, 131–45
Scott, Sir Walter, 136
Select Committee on Anatomy, 137–38, 140
sex, 28, 53, 76
sheepskin, 13, 22, 24, 32
Sheridan, Bridgette, 81
Sherwood, Kyle, 189–91
shrunken heads, 174, 175
"Siamese Twins," 3
signatures, 35; of bookbinders, 75

Simpson, Abigail, 135
slavery, 95, 104, 105, 106, 110–11
smallpox, 135
Smith, Bertram, 106
Snow, Mikel, 212, 216
Soap Lady, 62–65
Sorbonne, 198
Southern California Society for the History of Medicine, 10–11
Spain, 22
speculum, 50
spelling, 12 and *n*
Spurzheim, Johann, 122–23
squirrel skin, 71
SS, 175, 179, 181
Stanford University, 164; Stanford Medical History Center, 164, 166, 168
St. Edmundsbury Borough Council, 127
Stein, Harry, 175
Steinbeck, John, 207
Steiner, Tim, 187–88
St. John's Health Center, Santa Monica, 10
stolen books, Nazi, 171–73
suede, 155; *see also* ooze
Surgeons' Hall Museums, at the Royal College of Surgeons of Edinburgh, 132, 194
Surgeons' Square, 131, 134, 135, 136
Swetland, Luke, 11–12, 16, 41
Syracuse Daily Standard, 88
Syracuse Public Library, 88
Syracuse University Library, 88

Tabor, Stephen, 7–8, 9
tanning, 14, 15, 22–25, 67–77, 167; animal skin, 68–77; bating, 73; chrome method, 68, 70; fish, 74; French Revolution-era, 37–47; human skin, 67–77; liming process, 72–73; methods, 67–77; smell, 69; urine, 74–75; vegetable methods, 68, 70, 73, 74
tannins, 73, 75
tattoos, 23–24, 174–75, 185–92, 200; postmortem preservation of, 185–92
taxidermy, 17

Taylor, Telford, 181–82
Temple University, 103*n*
Te Papa, 195
text blocks, 26
Thompson, Lawrence S., 40
Topographische Anatomie des Menschen, see Pernkopf's *Atlas*
trichinosis, 49–51, 55, 56–57
tripe, 69
triple vocabulaire infernal, Le, 202
trypsin, 13
tuberculosis, 49, 50, 57, 151
Tullis, Jillian, 112
Tuskegee Syphilis Study, 111

United States Holocaust Memorial Museum, 177
University College of London, 138
University of Berlin, 163
University of California, Berkeley, 35–38, 46, 97; Bancroft Library, 35–38, 46
University of Cincinnati, 106
University of Edinburgh, 132, 133, 194; Anatomical Museum, 194
University of Notre Dame, 99–103; Hesburgh Library, 99–103
University of Paris, 84
University of Pennsylvania, 51, 52, 54, 58, 60, 62–63, 113
University of San Diego, 112
University of Southern California, 6, 169, 208, 211; anatomy program, 211–23; Keck School of Medicine of USC, 213; Norris Medical Library, 169
University of Southern Mississippi Libraries, 108
urine, 74–75
uterine vellum, 71

Vatinel, Sébastien, 203–205
vegetable tanning methods, 68, 70, 73, 74
vellum, 101, 198; Japanese, 108, 109; uterine, 71; *see also* cowhide; parchment

Verlaine, Paul, *Chair*, 200
Vesalius, Andreas, *Andreae Vesalii Bruxellensis . . . De humani corporis fabrica . . .*, 229
Vicq-d'Azyr, Félix, *Essai sur les lieux et les dangers des sépulture*, 229
Villeneuve, Pierre-Charles de, 41
Voltaire, 200

Wake Forest University, 191
Wales, 192
Walton, George, 147–59; *Narrative of the Life of James Allen, Alias George Walton, Alias Jonas Pierce, Alias James H. York, Alias Burley Grove the Highwayman*, 154–59, 229; skin used for books, 153–59
Warburton, Henry, 138, 140–41
war casualties, 4, 61–62
Ward, Alie, 218
Warren, Leonard, 59
Washington, George, 105, 154
Washington, Harriet, *Medical Apartheid*, 110, 111
watermarks, 35
Watson, Blake, 10
Watson, Brooks, 105
Webster, Noah, 12*n*
Wellcome, Henry, 96–98
Wellcome Collection, 91–92, 187
Wellcome Library, 128
Wellcome Trust, 97, 127
West Port Murders, 135, 137; *see also* Burke and Hare murders
whales, 13
Wheatley, John, 104, 105
Wheatley, Phillis, 104–10, 166*n*, 194; human skin copies, 106–10; *Poems on Various Subjects, Religious and Moral*, 105, 106–10, 229, 230
Wheatley, Susanna, 104, 105
Whitechapel murders, 90–91
Widener Library, at Harvard University, 164
Wiesel, Elie, 173

Wilson, Albert Monroe, 112–13
Wilson, Franklin T., 158
Win, Benjamin, 212
Wistar Institute, 62–63
women, 90, 162; Black authors, 104–10; childbirth, 79–84; corpses of murdered women exploited, 90–92; doctors, 84–85; health and reproduction, 50, 53, 79–84, 224, 227; hormonal imbalance, 224–25, 227; human skin books made from, 50–57, 67, 72–77, 85–86, 91, 199; midwives, 79–84; Red Barn murder, 115–30; Soap Lady, 62–65
Wood, Charles Erskine Scott, 207
wood pulp, 35
workhouses, 138, 141
World War I, 164, 177

World War II, 126, 164, 174, 177
Wyoming Valley, Pennsylvania, 11–12

Ximenes, Cardinal, 100

Yamashita, Warren, "Letter of Apology," 212–13
yellow fever, 63–64
Yonger, Prince, 95

Zaehnsdorf, Joseph, 108
Zamorano Club, 7–8
Zentral- und Landesbibliothek, 172, 173
Zürich, 189